Weight Training for Golf

for Golf

The Ultimate Guide

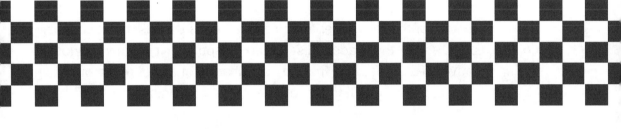

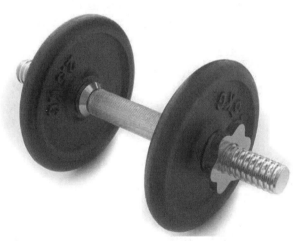

PW
PRICE WORLD
PUBLISHING

WEIGHT TRAINING FOR GOLF

Weight Training for Golf – The Ultimate Guide

Copyright © 2012 by Kai Fusser.

First Edition 2012

ISBN: 978-1932-54977-3

ISBN: 978-1936-91015-1 (ebook)

Library of Congress Control Number: 2011916301

Published by Price World Publishing

1300 W. Belmont Ave. Suite #20g

Chicago, IL 60657

All photos of exercises taken by
Jonathan Pears

For information about discounts for bulk purchases, please contact info@priceworldpublishing.com.

Printing by Cushing-Malloy, Inc.

Printed in the United States of America

10 9 8 7 6 5 4 3

Contents

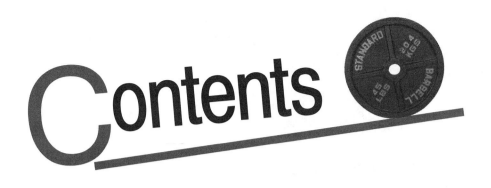

KAI FUSSER

Part 3

Part 4

Part 5

Praise for the author

"I STARTED TO work out with Kai at the end of 2009, because I felt after my rookie season on the LPGA I was lacking the strength and the fitness needed to be competitive on tour. I had always worked out in one way or another, but with Kai's systematic training programs everything started to make much more sense. I know the programs will help me get the most out of every session and that it will help me get to my peak performance.

While working out with Kai for the last 16 months, I have gained 25 yards off the tee and I am hitting my irons a club and a half further. I am much more consistent and I now have the strength to handle the deep rough we face on tour with no problems. Kai has taught me how to be more effortless and efficient thru his fitness regime and it has helped my game tremendously.

Kai continuously amazes me with his knowledge and his ways to motivate me to become the best athlete I can be. His passion, commitment and work-ethic is second to none, and I am very fortunate to have Kai on my team. He brings out the best in me, and I am sure he can do wonders for you too."

Anna Nordqvist,
LPGA Tour professional

"I HAVE BEEN following Kai and his work with professional women's golfers for a long time and I can see the difference he is making, a strong connection with the work he does and the results his athletes (players) achieve, both as golfers and human beings. As a coach, that is what you want to see.

Katarina Vangdal
Head Coach, Swedish Golf Team

WHEN I FIRST met Kai, I was playing full time on the LPGA Tour and I was in pretty good strength shape. I told him that my goal for working with him would be to not feel and move like a tank! Today I'm in the best shape of my life in so many ways. I feel like I have a different understanding on how the body works and how to use the muscles in a more efficient way due to the training that I have done with Kai. My swing is stronger now compared to when I played on the LPGA tour as I have worked on the smaller (stabilizing) muscles to match my big muscles. I have also increased distance with my driver from my active days on tour. My body does not feel like a tank any longer and I can move more gracefully even while being stronger. My endurance is also much better due to the interval training that we do instead of going out for long runs, it saves me a lot of time this way and my knees and hips thanks me for it.

Now as a swing coach I can use and explain movements in the swing much better to my students. When the students struggle with some movements in the swing, I just send them in to Kai. Then they understand and are able to create the movement I am asking for and at the same time get stronger and faster.

Kai's training is not only efficient but FUN and QUICK, what more can you ask for.

Charlotta Sorenstam
Director of Golf Operations, ANNIKA Academy
Certified Callaway Club Fitter
LPGA T&CP

I have been Annika's coach for over 20 years and have seen her grow from being a good Junior player to be the best in the world for several years in a row. Together we constantly worked on her swing and short game expecting nothing but perfection. Entering into a serious and well thought out fitness program with Kai in 2001 added another dimension to her game: new found strength, balance, and control helped to propel her game to the next and highest level.

Fast forward 10 years and now we are using the same proven combination of solid coaching and physical training for all our shared students, from the recreational player to aspiring Juniors to Professionals

Kai has made my job easier, the players have better body awareness and control and are able to better transfer my instructions into action.

Listen to him and you will improve your game!

Henri Reis

Acknowledgments

WRITING A BOOK takes a tremendous amount of effort and time. Your mind is constantly occupied with that project, and ideas come up at the strangest times, moments which sometimes will make you forget about the outside world. So if have neglected anyone in the last six months, please forgive me. I'm back now.

My heartfelt thanks to my beautiful wife, Tina, who I single-mindedly chased after, starting in fifth grade. (You, too, will learn the benefits of persistence and determination in this book.) Tina and I share the same passion for fitness and nutrition; it's our life and we do it together. You will see her demonstrate the stretching exercises. Thanks to my wonderful daughter, Tess, who is a cheerleader at Florida State and followed my workout programs — she is ripped! And my equally wonderful son, Tim, a soccer player with big plans and the determination to reach his goals.

I want to thank all of my athletes. I may have taught them how to build a perfect body for their sport, but they have taught me so much more.

My deepest thanks to Annika, the best student I could ever dream of having. I have learned so much from her — her vision, preparation and execution is incredible; that's why she is the best. Also, to Anna Nordqvist, the girl who never stops, is always up for a challenge, always hungry for the new and better. I'm certain we'll continue to hear a lot about Anna in the future. Thanks, too, to Karen Stupples, the power woman. Watch her drive! And to Minea Blomqvist, a young mother juggling it all and getting back to the top; Graeme McDowell, the nicest pro I have ever had the pleasure to meet on tour, and Shannon and Simin, my juniors who keep me on the up and up and always bring fun into the gym.

My thanks, too, to all the non-golfing athletes who contributed to my understanding of movement, including Grant Hill, Eddie Cheever, Darin

Shapiro, Raimi Merritt, and Will Asher — how exceptional they are.

I would also like to thank the crew at the ANNIKA Academy: Henri, with whom it is so fun to share students with, Charlotta, the strongest Swede I know, together we can fix any swing; and Mark, who keeps a secret tape of my swing on the V-1 system; Pam who runs the show and keeps everyone in line, I know she feels like she's herding goats sometimes; Jackson whom I drive nuts with all my requests. We deal with each other every day while running the best golf school in the world, always with love and respect.

Thanks to all the professionals who have taught me. Some of them are now my good friends and some I have never met. These include Dr. Christian Haid, the best when it comes to physics and biomechanics, who really opened my eyes and whom I'm grateful to have as a friend; Chuck Wolf, another movement specialist; Dr. Steve Chaney, my go-to source for research and invaluable nutritional insights; Dr. Michael Colgan, whose writings I love and whom I hope to meet some day; Juan Carlos Santana, Paul Check and Mark Verstegen for their books and seminars — these guys have it figured out.

To Rob Price, my publisher, my thanks for taking me on and dealing with my "Germ-lish" German English.

Thanks to Bob Ferguson and Gregg Cochlan for introducing me to The Pacific Institute and its teachings, where they make using the brain fun; to Lou Tice — it was a honor to meet you; you can change the world!

I thank everyone that has walked through my gym and all the guests of the ANNIKA Academy. Everyone is special and has something to teach. Thanks for rewarding me by reaching your goals.

A special thanks to my parents who are still super-active in their seventies — thanks for raising me to be a good boy, Mom, thanks for feeding me so well, and, Dad, thanks for making me that dumbbell 40-something years ago.

Thanks to our creator for giving us the freedom to make our own decisions.

Introduction

In 2010, I was asked to address more than 200 trainers at a conference in Orlando to tell my story of how I became a successful personal trainer. That's when it really hit home how long I have been experimenting, trying to improve physical performance.

I asked my dad if he could find the dumbbell that I had begun using at the age of about six or seven. He had fabricated it at his workplace back then, wrapping it in electrical tape to make it look nicer. That was 43 years ago.

I also remember the "Expander," a hot workout tool in those days. The springs were forever getting caught in my hair when doing exercises behind the head. I am convinced that is the sole reason I have that shiny, bald spot on the back of my head today.

Over the years I ventured into many different sports: soccer, sailing, bodybuilding, boxing, motorcycling, waterskiing and more, always with a relentless urge to perfect my every movement.

Many people are afraid of getting older. Me, I love it, as every day we experience something new; we learn and hopefully get a little smarter. What I have learned over the years has been an accumulation of trying — doing as well as studying, whereas the trying and doing has certainly had a bigger impact.

I also learned a lot from being around the great athletes from different sports I have worked with, like Annika, Graeme McDowell, Grant Hill, Darin Shapiro, Eddie Cheever and more. They all found and developed very special abilities in their respective sports. Those special abilities are ultimately universal in the world of top athletes. Belief, consistency and determination is what got them to where they are; nothing came for free; everything had to be earned.

This is what it will take to reach your goal, whether it be to hit it an extra 10 yards, break 90, win your club championship or even the US Open.

WEIGHT TRAINING FOR GOLF

I met Annika in 2001 when she was looking for a trainer in Orlando. I hadn't the first clue about golf, having never played it. That lack of golf knowledge turned out to be a blessing for me, as I had no preconception about how a workout for golfers should ideally be. At that time, I had trained many water skiers and wake boarders, and had competed in water skiing myself for many years. These athletes were tough, very tough. Their sports require tremendous strength, balance and body control, so they needed workouts designed to handle the stresses on their body.

My background in engineering and physics gave me a very good understanding of the mechanics of the golf swing and I could see the biomechanical improvements necessary in order to improve it.

During the first training session with Annika, I realized very quickly that she was a true athlete in every sense of the word. She wanted to improve her game by becoming more athletic and didn't hold back. I began using the same workouts with her that I had implemented for my skiers and boarders, with some variations. She took very well to it.

After about four months of training, Annika had gained over 20 yards with her driver while at the same time improving her accuracy. She went on to win thirteen tournaments in the 2002 season, a truly incredible feat.

In 2003 Annika had the strength to compete against the men at Colonial; from tee to green, she kept up with the best of them. She developed a swing that, from a biomechanical and physics standpoint, is one of the most efficient, reliable and healthy swings. A swing that for anybody, Men or Women can be used long term, into a very high playing age as it also is very forgiving on the body.

Back in 2003, Annika and I began exploring the concept of the total golfer. This combination of the swing, course management, fitness and nutrition helped Annika to reach her goals, begin planning her future Academy and, just four years later see her dream realized when they broke ground. Annika's passion for golf and fitness has also led her to found the ANNIKA® Foundation which interest is the development of a healthy lifestyle for kids through fitness and nutrition (www.AnnikaFoundation.org).

At the ANNIKA Academy™ we now get many guests and students from beginners to scratch players going through our two- and three-day programs, which include swing and short game coaching, club fitting and course management, as well as fitness training and nutrition education. We treat the game of golf as an accumulation of all those aspects, the same aspects that helped Annika to become one of the best to ever play the game. The coaches are Henri Reis, Annika's coach for over 25 years, Charlotta Sorenstam, an LPGA player for 15 years, Mark Bereza, coach and certified club fitter and me, Annika's trainer for more than 10 years.

My gym at the Academy is only fifty feet from the practice area and driving range, and I can see every student's swing from my window, which really helps with the integration of the swing and fitness. What we as a team have learned working so closely together is that almost all of the "swing faults" also show up in certain exercises in the gym, which means that many of these swing faults can be fixed in the gym much quicker then on the range.

When practicing on the range, the feedback you receive is very minimal, mostly focused on the ball flight, to give an indication of what occurred during the swing. Each player concentrates on the ball, ensuring they make contact with the ball every time, no matter what or how (often while compromising the health of their body). Everything happens very quickly.

In the gym, we can take certain movements of the swing, perform them in front of the mirror at slow speed with some resistance for better feedback without the ball. In this way, each student can concentrate, feel and learn at a much higher rate than when on the range. That is one of the great advantages of working out: improving your movements to improve

your swing quickly, and save you much time and frustration on the range.

As another benefit, in the gym the student can also become stronger, gain greater control, power and endurance, all benefits of proper weight training.

Admittedly, what *Weight Training for Golf – The Ultimate Guide* can provide to improve your technique is not as extensive as what I could accomplish with you in person at the ANNIKA Academy™ in Orlando, Florida, as there is nothing like seeing someone first-hand as they move in order to correct, improve and ultimately perfect that movement through hands-on training. However, this book is a terrific way for you to begin through self-training to improve your swing.

My goal in *Weight Training for Golf – The Ultimate Guide* is to teach you these very same principles and workout techniques that I have used successfully over the years with many golfers, from recreational players to junior players and even professionals.

The text is designed to be as simple as possible, without delving into research, as much of that can be found in my list of recommended reading and other references, as well as my website, www.kaifusser.com. The aim of this book is to be a handy guide, not a scientific manual.

KAI FUSSER

I teach biomechanically sound, efficient and safe movements to learn how to control your body best during a static state, acceleration and deceleration. What you then do with what you have learned is up to you, but ideally you would incorporate those principles into your swing.

Understand that there are no miracle exercises or workouts, also this book does not include all exercises in existence, the difference is the way the exercises are performed! and this is what you will learn.

In *Weight Training for Golf – The Ultimate Guide*, I will teach you the same concepts that I have used to help players at all different levels, from rank beginners to top professionals to build strength and improve their swing. There are right ways to do weight training for golf and wrong ways. When done right, you will love the benefits it gives you both on and off the course.

To better illustrate how important it is to differentiate between the right way to train and the wrong way, here is a story the photographer for this book, an avid skydiver, shared with me. During one of his sky diving courses, there was a fellow skydiving student who was a serious body builder, about five feet nine inches tall and weighing about 220 pounds. Now, when you jump, obviously you need to know where the rip cord is in order to deploy your parachute. It's located behind you, along your lower back. Now, all the students including the bodybuilder knew where their rip cords were. However, on his first solo jump, when he jumped out of the plane and it came time to pull the cord, this bodybuilder's muscles were so big that they got in the way — he was so tight that he could not reach the cord to open his chute! Luckily for him, his instructor was nearby, spotted his difficulty and reached in and pulled it for him.

I call this the wrong training for your sport. With *Weight Training for Golf – The Ultimate Guide*, I'll give you the proper tools for effective weight training so that you're never left hanging in the breeze.

These were the days:

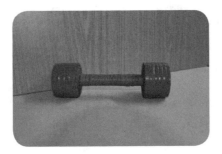

Here you see the DB that my dad had made for me, ca. 1968 (yes the electrical tape is new)

Do you remember the expander? if yes you are probably at least as old as I am.

1979, this was in my early days travelling the world as a sailor. The first officer on that ship was all into sports and he took us youngsters under his wing, I owe him much of my love for fitness. We built a gym in the hull at the bottom of the ship and after a hard day at sea would go to work out which kept us out of trouble (for the most part).

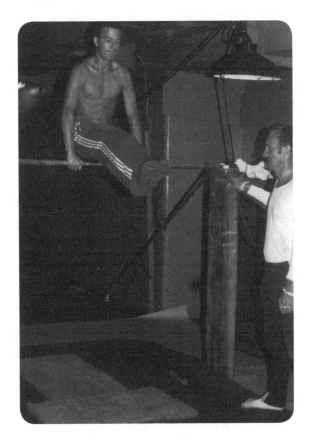

The Scope of This Book

THIS BOOK IS intended to be a "workout guide" more so than a scientific publication.

It covers exercises and workouts for a wide variety of applications and users ranging from the total beginner to the professional golfer. Whichever category you see yourself in will determine the time, effort, grade of difficulty and intensity you put into your workouts.

It can range from just doing some of the stretches to picking a few strength or swing fault exercises. Or you can do the full program from the Building And Learning phase through the Power Phase into the In Season Phase, which will take much time, determination and consistency.

My intention is that you understand the connection between golf and weight training, that you learn how to work out correctly and safely, that you improve both your golf and your health, that you enjoy the journey and value the benefits, and, most of all, that you have fun.

Many topics in this book warrant a book individually — just think of nutrition, for example. It is a very big subject which you have to deal with every day of your life, making the right decisions with every meal. I have tried to keep it simple and invite you to educate yourself more on the topics that interest you and can make a difference in your life by including some recommended reading on different subjects. While certainly not a complete list, it is a good start. You will also find more information, updates, resources and news on my website, www.kaifusser.com.

There is also a little secret in this book: that anybody can benefit from the principles and exercises contained in this book, no matter which sport they play. I use the same programs for my water skiers and wake boarders, or race car drivers, or NBA players — it's just that the emphasis and intensity changes with their respective needs. At the end you want to build a perfect body and use it as you wish, may it be for yard work or golf or an MMA fight.

Part 1

Why Weight Training for Golf

IT IS NOT that long ago that weight training was thought of as detrimental to the golf swing as well as for putting; it was said that weight training will get golfers "too tight" and "too bulky," that it will take away the ability to move with flexibility, and that golf is an endurance sport, not a strength sport.

When I started working with Annika in 2001, the fitness training for golfers mainly consisted of some cardio training, some abdominal training and lots of stretching. Annika (along with Tiger on the men's side) has been instrumental in changing that forever. She has demonstrated that weight training can have a big positive effect and most every professional golfer is now doing some form of it.

Now, I agree that the wrong approach to weight training can hurt your ability to move your body effectively for golf. Looking at a bodybuilder full of muscles and bulk, it is easy to see how the wrong weight training can bind up the body and its ability to move freely and efficiently. At the same time, a bodybuilder is not interested in movement but in "display" and for that purpose his style of training is just fine.

The problem we see in most of the gyms today is that most everyone is working out by "body building principles" even though they are not body builders.

What you also have to realize is that you need to prepare your body for the rigors of golf. Most amateurs swing their drivers with almost their full energy output. Add the many other swings, bending and turning at high speeds, accelerating, decelerating and controlling the club head while it's moving at 100 miles per hour and you start to see that golf is not as easy on our bodies as one would think. For your body to handle that stress, especially if you want to play into a high age, it needs to be prepared by strengthening your whole physical system: bones, muscles, ligaments and tendons; also by learning to move efficiently and being able to control the forces applied.

In the upcoming chapters, I will go to great lengths to explain how to do weight training the right way, and it is important that you follow these recommendations in order to achieve your goals.

Now here is what you can expect with the right weight training:

Strength: determines the ability to move an object (in your case, the golf club) or your body.

Speed: critical for the production of power as it is an exponential factor.

Power: the result of mass, strength and speed, and is a major factor in achieving distance as well as getting the ball out of the rough.

Range of Motion: the ability to move your limbs and torso in their intended range of motion; for golf it is important to develop a good range of motion in your shoulders, hips and spine.

Stability: the ability to stabilize your body during still stand (static stability during address position and putting) as well as movement (dynamic stability during acceleration and deceleration during the swing phase); stability is dependent on strength, balance and control of speed and rhythm.

Balance: the ability to control your body during static and dynamic movement.

Endurance: the ability to perform at a desired level over a certain amount of time. There is muscular and cardiovascular endurance required in golf — you need to be able to repeat highly skilled moves over a long period of time, which requires more muscular endurance; the endurance level is also dependent on how efficient your movements are.

Efficiency: the ability to perform a movement, propel yourself or an object in the most efficient way without wasting energy or creating unnecessary stress on your body.

Protection: the ability to protect your body from the stress created in your joints and soft tissue during the swing and putting; this is dependent on the strength of the stabilizing muscles in the joints, the correct movement patterns, and efficiency.

Longevity: the ability to use your body at its highest performance level for as long as possible. For my athletes, I call that their shelf life. It is the culmination of all of the above. **What you teach your body and how you prepare it determines what you will have to work with in the future.**

As you can see, all of the benefits that you want to gain through weight training are dependent on each other; therefore, the training has to be done with all of them in mind.

I can promise you from my experience that if you train right — with the right quality, intensity and quantity, and with the right support of nutrition and rest — that your body will perform at the level you expect it to and beyond.

This program will redesign and build up every aspect of your body needed for a perfectly functional system, starting with strengthening your connective tissue to protect your joints, learning to use your core for power, control and protection, and learning to move at the highest efficiency rate while increasing your endurance and longevity.

Besides the obvious benefits from weight training for your golf game, you will also be healthier, feel better, look better and be stronger, have more confidence, increase your metabolism and more.

Enjoy your workouts and reap the benefits.

Women versus Men

Now, ONE MIGHT say this is a very obvious point to make, but I would like to point out some differences when it comes to training, getting stronger and more powerful. I work with more female athletes than male, even though I have been very successful with guys like Graeme McDowell (PGA), Grant Hill (NBA) or Darin Shapiro (Wake Boarding).

First I need to say, hats off to the ladies — sorry, guys, but they're tougher than you are, especially when it comes to handling pain. There is much less crying about soreness or complaining that "this is too hard...." Clearly, there is reason why your bodies bear babies; we guys sure could not handle it.

Many times I am asked by women: will I get too big or bulk up when I do heavy weight training? Rest assured that when the training is done correctly, as described in this book, this will not happen. Plus you lack the hormonal setup that would make you too muscular.

Annika did 300-pound squats, 160-pound bench presses and 15 pull ups and it did not have a negative effect on her appearance (but sure had a positive effect on her performance).

Women are almost as strong in the legs as men but their biggest disparity is in the upper body, especially the connection between the arms and the torso, which are the chest muscles and the back muscles (mainly lattisimus dorsi), as well as the arms.

You have probably seen some guys on the range who can muscle a golf ball a decent distance by using their arms only. Even though this is not very efficient, they still can get away with it. For women this does not work as well, because your arms and shoulders are simply not strong enough.

As you will see in this book, there is much attention given to building upper body strength through exercises like chest presses, push ups, pull ups and other pulling and pushing ex-

KAI FUSSER

ercises. This will give you the strength and control needed to produce the power necessary to hit the ball longer but also to be able to get out of the thickest rough.

At the same time, you want to learn to use the strength of your legs and hips to build power and stability, as well as how to transfer that power through your midsection and upper body to the club (and this is true for Men as well).

Another difference is the ability to load and unload your body. For us men, it is more natural to take advantage of the elastic strain energy we can produce during a rotational or up and down movement.

Compare a girl and a boy throwing a rock. What you will see most of the time is that the girl will pause during the backside of the rotation (swing) which leads to the loss of all built up energy created by the motion of going back. Now, the forward movement has to start from scratch to accelerate again. That's very inefficient. Meanwhile, the boy will have a seamless transition between the backward and forward movement essentially even increasing the built up energy. Think of snapping a towel or cracking a whip.

This loading and unloading just has to be learned. There are great exercises that can be done to help this, like medicine ball throws and performing rotational exercises with continuous acceleration.

An advantage women have over men is that they generally swing with a smoother rhythm and less erratic movements, which leads to better stability and accuracy.

Recreational vs. Professional

How Much and How Hard

How WOULD A recreational or amateur player work out differently than a professional player?

Now, that is really up to the individual. Obviously, the higher your goals are, the better and more intensely you will want to work out.

For golf, I would say that about five full workouts a week will cover all the workout needs of a pro, provided that they are of high quality and the right intensity. Additional to that would be good warm-ups before practice and play, as well as some stretching and recovery exercises.

For a recreational player, two workouts a week can be of great value, again provided that the quality and intensity is right.

While the professional players hardly have a choice — in order to become the best they can be getting the right amount and quality of workout in is critical — for the recreational player, it's just a matter of where he wants to be. But I would say that three to four workouts a week are sufficient.

What you need to realize is that the difference between doing three versus four workouts a week or four versus five workouts a week is not that great, as you will not get a linear increase in results for each extra workout. That means that the difference between four and five workouts might amount to as little as a five percent gain.

Now that five percent gain can make a huge difference for a professional as the separation between pros is mostly minute, but for a recreational player that extra workout may not give you enough payoff, considering the amount of effort required.

When Annika was at her strongest, around 2004 and 2005, we worked out four to five days a week. At that point, in order for her to gain any further strength, we would have had to add another day and go up even higher in intensity. However, this would gain her maybe a few percentage points stronger, but the extra time and the possibility for injury or overtraining did not make sense. Instead, we concentrated on perfecting her movement and efficiency while keeping her strength at the same level.

So it is a simple equation: the higher your goals are, the more you want to put into your workout, bearing in mind that the curve of gains will flatten out (plateau) the more workouts you do per week, with the risk of overtraining in the worst case.

Children and Juniors

I AM OFTEN asked how early a child can start working out. My answer is as soon as they can comprehend. The question more to the point is: what does a workout for a child look like? Much is dependent upon the child's biological age, meaning the mental and physical development level of the child.

Supervision and the right teaching are the keys. As a parent, I would suggest seeking help from a professional with experience working with young kids to get them started on the workout process.

I think it is important to instill a good work ethic early on in childhood. If children learn to take care of their bodies at a young age, it will feel normal and become routine at a later age. I have seen teenagers who have been playing tournament golf for some time and are reluctant to work out. They may not see the value of working out as they have been successful until then without it.

This can be a problem down the road in terms of performance, but, more important, in terms of health. Too often the very young golfer has been over-trained by hitting countless balls, as they are very flexible but lack the stability and strength within their flexibility range; the joints are unprotected and at some point the wear will take its toll. So workout or "preparation" for the stresses of the sport has to go hand in hand with the skills practice.

I have trained kids as young as seven years old. A workout at that age takes a maximum of 20 to 30 minutes and mainly consists of exercises with body weight or *very light* resistance from dumbbells, cables, medicine balls or rubber bands, making sure to teach the right form and movement patterns. A certain amount of play (fun) needs to be included to keep the child engaged.

A full three- or four-day workout can begin at age 13 to 14 for girls, and 14 to 15 for boys, initially limiting the workout time to 30 to 45 minutes, and gradually increasing to a maximum of one hour, starting with

KAI FUSSER

light weights until there is absolute perfect form, including the ability to engage the core to protect the spine. By the age of 16 to 17 for girls and 17 to 18 for the boys, they can be working out at full capacity in terms of time and intensity, again, supervision is the key.

I work with several young AJGA players (in addition to other sports) and I can tell you it is an absolute pleasure: the level of commitment and dedication is amazing, and seeing the results is very rewarding for both the athlete and myself.

EQuipment and Workout Schemes

THERE ARE ALL kinds of different workout equipment available today. Just when you think they have invented it all, some new piece will show up on the market, always the best and only one that you need to reach your fitness dreams. This is also true when it comes to all those group classes and DVD workouts. There are many people who are addicted to certain equipment or classes. What you need to realize is that overdoing even the best workout method will lead to staleness, imbalance and often injury.

You may hear from a Spinning, Step, Yoga, Cross Fit or other class instructor that all you need to do is come to his or her class five days a week and you will reach your fitness goal. While each of these classes has its purpose and upsides, it is also easy to overdo it; none of them will take care of it all.

Your body is very multidimensional and can move in countless ways and that's how we need to train it.

Also, some classes are built around high speeds and impact. While this can work well for getting more powerful and in shape, it is also very stressful on your system, especially on the joints, therefore, they should only be taken for a certain time period (four to six weeks) in order to give the body some rest. You also need to do some buildup and support exercises to prepare the body for that high stress.

The human body has been designed from the beginning to do two things: propel itself and/or propel an object, think of walking or jumping, or lifting a cup of coffee or a suitcase. In your case, as a golfer you propel the club when you lift it, and propel your body when you rotate and shift your weight — all that while freestanding and controlling the movement as much as possible. All this movement is also gravity dependent. So what you need to do most in order to get stronger, faster, more balanced, etc., is move yourself or a weight (or both) from point A to point B, ideally unrestricted and in absolute control.

Here is a list of the most common exercise equipment and my experience and opinion of it (I may not make many friends with this one):

Machines (i.e., leg press, chest press, curl, Smith, etc.)

Hurt yourself

Stay away from them! (except in some rare rehabilitation cases.) They will hurt you in the long run! As you are sitting in the machine, maybe even buckled up, most parts of your body will be shut out of the movement. The machine will do all the stabilizing for you while you isolate the moving muscles. That means that your primary movers (e.g., the quadriceps in the leg extension) will get stronger but most of the stabilizing muscles surrounding your joints (i.e., the knees, ankles and hips) will not get equally stronger. Now you go out hiking or play tennis, take a bad step and your strong quadriceps pulls against the weak stabilizers in your knee and guess what will give in? You can either pull some muscles or, worse, your ligaments can be damaged. Also, the machines can produce some grinding in the joints as they are not able to move freely while the movement is guided by the machine. In addition it will not teach your nervous system how to stabilize and balance as the machine does that for you.

Your Own Body

Propel yourself

Perfect! You always have it with you. And it is free. Countless exercises can be done with your own body weight for strengthening, speed, balance and endurance.

Free Weights (e.g., dumbbells, barbells, kettle bells, medicine balls)

Propel an object

Still the best way to learn how to move an object against gravity, accelerating and decelerating it while staying in control just like your golf club. Use these to build strength, stability, balance, speed and power.

Cable Pull

Propel yourself while increasing resistance

I love the cable pull! You can do countless strengthening and rotational exercises on it. Your body can be loaded with resistance from all different angles and you have to figure out how to stay in control at the same time. Many parts of the swing can be practiced perfectly on it as well.

Rubber Bands

Movement and Stretching

Although I do not prefer rubber bands to build strength (you are not working against gravity and they are not as efficient as working with weights), they have their place and are great for performing movements with speed and for gradual increasing and decreasing resistance during rotational moves. I also prefer them for stretching instead of using a solid object; great take along as an exercise alternative while travelling or at home.

Physio Ball

Balance and strength

Great tool for countless exercises, including developing core strength, balance and control; easy to use at home. (make sure to inspect the ball before use, you don't want it to come apart while being on it)

Balance Board (various models, I prefer the Indoboard™)

One of the best ways to increase balance and control, as well as strengthening your joint and stabilizing muscles. Most standing exercises can and should at some level be done on a balance board.

Jump Rope

One of my favorites

Great for cardiovascular and speed training; requires coordination between the hands and feet while also being relaxed. Also a great tool for warming up before play or workout.

Treadmill

Too many of them

If you really need to run, go outside! While the treadmill is running, all you are doing is trying to keep up with the belt. What athlete merely wants to keep up? You want to set the pace. The only way to use a treadmill is to turn the motor off and push the belt. We use them extensively like that, as it builds super strength in the legs as well as in the upper body, all while minimizing the impact on your joints.

Elliptical Machine

Way too many of them

I am not a big fan of them as they are almost perpetual — get on it and enjoy the ride while watching your favorite show. I am not saying they are all bad, but the return on the time you invest on it is very minimal. When you work out, you want 100 percent back of what you put in.

Stationary Bike

Still one of the better machines

Great for knee strength and cardio sessions, especially for high intensity sprints. Choose the upright over the recumbent, and turn that fan off!

Upper Body Ergo Meter (bicycle for your arms)

Another one of my favorites

If it has one, move the chair out of the way, stand up and use your whole body. Great for the arms, shoulders and for high intensity sprints. Learn how to keep your grip, arms and shoulders relaxed while producing a maximum amount of energy (I have been able to bring many high level athletes to their knees on that machine).

Part 2

Be the Best You Can Be

" BE THE BEST YOU CAN BE "

TO REACH YOUR 100% POTENTIAL EACH OF THE 5 PIE's NEED TO BE FILLED iN 100%
HAS ANYBODY EVER REACHED 100% OF THEIR FULL POTENTIAL ? NOBODY CAN ANSWER
THAT QUESTION. ALL YOU CAN DO is OPTIMIZE EACH AREA AS BEST AS POSSIBLE WITH
ALL YOU KNOW, ALL YOU LEARN
AND ALL THE HELP YOU CAN GET.

PHYSICAL TRAINING

NUTRITION + HEALTH

TECHNICAL TRAINING

REST + RECUPERATION

FOCUS + MIND

KAT FUSSER

WHAT DOES IT take to become the best you can be?

Over the years I have worked with and watched athletes who reached the point of becoming the best they could be (with what we know).

What I have learned is that it takes 100 percent optimization in the five areas around the sport, which are:

1. **Focus and mental strength**: you have to know where you want to go, otherwise you will never get there. Have an understanding what it takes to get there, set clear goals, and take the most direct path to reach your goals without any distraction. Requires

mental training, preparation and application.

2. **Technical training**: have the right coach, learn the right technique. Requires optimum and efficient practice. Use the right equipment; get the right help from technology.

3. **Physical training**: have the right trainer; optimize your strength, power, flexibility, endurance and movement patterns; train for peaking, train for protection and longevity

4. **Nutrition and health**: ensure the right quality and quantity for performance, recuperation and health; avoid forced breaks through a healthy lifestyle

5. **Rest and recuperation**: get enough quality sleep (8-10 hours a day); optimize recuperation from training and play; get mental rest; optimize the right time off from your sport.

Think of each of these five areas as equally valuable, worth 20 percent apiece to total 100 percent potential. If you are not reaching 100 percent optimization in each area, you are missing out on the possible collective total, which means you are missing out on your full potential.

I recommend you evaluate and adjust each of these five areas on an ongoing basis, get help from your team, such as your coach and trainer, to identify any deficiencies.

The Quality of Your Workout – Perfect Training Generates Perfect Movements

The quality of your exercises performed is the biggest determining factor of your success.

What you need to understand is: **what your body does most often is what it will repeat,** and that is especially critical when it comes to training for golf as this is a sport that is build on highly intricate movements — each slight variation will result in a different outcome. The swing is nothing else than an accumulation of different movements controlled by the laws of physics. If your shoulders are off by three degrees and your arms by two degrees, the ball flight will be drastically different from your norm. Or you will compensate with "bad" movements to make sure you will hit the ball.

This means that you need to strive to do every exercise perfectly and identically every single time, so your body learns and therefore is able to repeat. This also means that you want to concentrate on every single repetition. I like to say that, instead of doing a set of eight repetitions, do a set of eight single repetitions, each being a single unit done to perfection.

What you usually see in the gym is mindless lifting and moving (often while the mind is occupied watching

TV), which is fine for burning some calories and getting fitter but it will not contribute much to teaching, learning and repeating. If golf is your chosen sport, then you know that it is a constant learning process. After all, you would not line up eight balls and hit them quickly, one after the other, without any thought or concentration, right?

This is one reason why you don't want to work out for more than one hour at a time. Your concentration level will break down. You must remain alert and concentrate. Perfect training makes for perfect movements.

I would also recommend not wearing gloves, as there are many receptors in your hands and fingers which send signals to your brain and nervous system as soon as you touch something. These signals are important in order for your body to respond at 100 percent capacity.

Warm Up Before Workout, Practice and Play

Warming up before any strenuous activity is very important. First, it is your best protection against injury. Second, it is the best way to prepare your nervous system for the upcoming demand of any high coordination exercise, including the swing.

Warming up means elevating the blood flow in your muscles through some controlled movements to prepare the muscles to react quickly to the demand of the exercises, mainly the stabilizing muscles of the joints.

Your stabilizing muscles surrounding the joints are responsible for protecting the limbs from going too far into the range of motion where the ligaments would have to take over the stabilization, which would create extra stress on the joint. The ligaments are attached closer to the joint than the muscles, which creates poor leverage and therefore more stress on all the connective tissue. This could result in stretched or torn ligaments either through one severe pull or through multiple repetitive pulls. So, it is important to incorporate every joint in the warmup, starting from the bigger muscles, like the legs, as they need longer to warm up than the smaller muscles, like the shoulders.

The warmup should be dynamic yet with a low impact on the joints, Start with a bike or light running on a treadmill or in place for three to five minutes. After that, you can progress into some moves like rope jumping, jumping jacks or knee-ups for two to three minutes, which require more coordination. Last, get more joint-specific with some ankle, hip, spine, shoulder and head rotations. Overall, a good warmup will take you about eight to ten minutes.

I personally do not see much value in stretching **before** a workout or play. Unless the muscles are really warmed up they will not "let go" anyway, and you will end up pulling on your tendons and ligaments. Plus, you want to prepare your body for a "dynamic" range of motion, not a "static" range of motion, hence we focus on a dynamic movement warmup versus static stretching. There are endless debates on the pros and cons of static stretching before a workout (and endless inconclusive studies). In my many years of training, I have yet to discover any value in doing it.

If you feel the need to stretch before your workout, I will not stop you, but just make sure you are warmed up thoroughly.

When it comes to practicing your swing and playing, I would strongly suggest you warm up at a minimum as described above. You may be embarrassed to jump around on the range but, believe me, you are the smart one. You can even do it at home if your commute to the range is not too long. The swing is a fairly violent move, especially for amateurs whose moves are very inefficient, and the forces in the joints can be very high, especially in the spine and the shoulders, so your stabilizing muscles had better be ready from the first swing onward.

I would also add some golf-specific exercises before practice or play,

depending on what you are working on in your swing. Pick one or two Swing Fault Exercises (from "Swing Fault Exercises" chapter) which will help to stimulate and prepare your nervous system accordingly.

My pro players warm up for at least 20 to 30 minutes before playing, as they understand the value of it. Anna Nordqvist often complained when we first began working together that she didn't feel completely ready until the third or fourth hole during her tournament rounds. When you consider that those two holes each round that she needed just to warm up accounted for nearly ten percent of the tournament total, that is not a good situation! We then came up with a 30-minute warmup routine that included pushups, lunges, squats, hammer curls and various rotational exercises. It wasn't long before she found herself ready on the first hole.

Some of my pros now even slot in a full workout before playing. Annika in particular loved working out before a round, even before major ones like the US Open or when she played the men at the Colonial. It made her feel loose and connected at the same time, and it also took the edge off a little and provided her with a good outlet to get away from the hustle of the tournament and release some stress.

Progressions – Constant Improvement

Progressions are very important in anything you do; otherwise, your body as well as your mind will get too comfortable and that's when your progress comes to a standstill. After all, the purpose of learning, training and practicing is to improve on your current state of abilities, not to remain static.

Your body is set up with a great tool for that: it's your defense mechanism, the constant urge for your system to protect and adapt. Basically your system will adapt to the demands you put on it. In the case of learning, if you ask your body to do a certain move often enough, it will react and do it at some point. It may take 50 times or even 5000 times, provided that you are willing to learn and know what to change. (That is also true when learning the wrong moves!)

In the case of gaining a physical trait like getting stronger muscles or improving your range of motion, your body will adapt the same way, to the demands you put on it. This means that you need to recognize when a movement or a load on your body gets too easy so as not to get stuck at that level.

With each exercise listed in this book, you will find a reference to which progressions can be applied. Here are the forms of progressions in the right order that you can deploy in order to move into the right direction toward your goals.

1. Learn the initial movement to perfection

All the principles of the right training have to be adhered to, good stance with slightly bent knees, straight axis, control out of the core and power flow (as explained in the upcoming chapters). Only after you know that the movement is perfect and you are comfortable with it, is it time to progress.

2. Add resistance

Adding resistance is the main factor in getting stronger, increasing the load on the muscles which triggers a signal to get stronger in order to adapt to the higher demand. This will also increase strength in our connective tissue, which will be needed when we increase speed. Increase the free weights, the weight on the cable or use a stronger rubber band.

3. Decrease stability

Decreasing stability will increase your balance and also build stronger stabilizing muscles. This can also be done parallel to adding resistance but not simultaneously, so don't add resistance and reduce stability at the same time during one exercise. You decrease stability by doing an exercise with the feet closer together or on one foot, standing or holding on to a balance board or even closing your eyes.

4. Increase speed

Increasing speed will have the biggest impact on your ability to produce power, therefore you want to learn how to produce speed but also learn how to control it. But speed will also put more stress on your body, mainly the connective tissue around the joints. So only after you have gone through the progressions above should you start to add speed. Speed also requires rhythm. This is very important especially for the golf swing as you should have a gradual increase of speed throughout your swing without any speed "spikes" along the way. This will lead to a gradual increase of power that is easier to stabilize and control (think of Annika's or Ernie Els's swing).

You can add speed to some full body exercises as well as rotational ones. Within the rotational exercises you want to duplicate the same rhythm as in your swing as closely as possible to learn the loading and unloading of the body as well as the right timing of the engagement of your abs during the movement.

Periodization

Periodization of workouts for performance is important for mainly two reasons.

First, you need to understand that strength, power, endurance, etc., have to be build in phases and that it takes time to reach your strongest level. Once reached you can only keep that level for a certain amount of time, when trained right — I would say about six to eight weeks. After that you need to start letting off and give your body some rest in order to prevent overtraining and injury.

Now, rest does not mean that you completely stop working out for a long period of time. (I would say that you can totally rest for about two weeks with no worries as it takes four to six weeks before your muscles start to weaken.) But you want to get away from any heavy and fast exercises. After the rest period, you can start again with the building and learning phase, or before that enjoy your newly gained strength and movement abilities for a while and venture into some other sports that you always wanted to try or improve on.

Second, if you play competitive golf and have a tournament season, you want to determine when you want to peak and then design the workout program where you will finish with the power phase about one to two weeks before that time and then enter into the in-season phase. That is important as you should not be in your hardest workout phase during the height of your competition season, which would just take too much energy.

For my tour players, the periodization looks like this:

Mid-November to end of January:
Building and learning phase

February to mid-April:
Strength phase

Mid-April to end of May:
Power phase

June to September:
In-season phase

October to mid-November:
Rest phase

During the long in-season phase, most of the players try not to play more than three tournaments in a row, which gives them an off tournament week every four weeks. During that off week we will do two or three "hard" workouts, consisting of a mix of heavy exercises from the strength and power phase, therefore, they will be able to keep their strength and power at a high level during that four-month period.

Reps, Weight, Speed, Range of Motion

In the exercise chapter, you will find a column with each exercise explaining the range of reps, speed and amount of weight recommended. In the programs section, you will find the more exact number depending on the workout phase you are in.

Always remember that any exercise has to be performed perfectly before you introduce any progressions like adding weight or speed.

1. Reps:

There are big debates on how many reps are right. In my opinion you can find the best explanation on that topic in Dr. Michael Colgan's book, "The New Power Program."

I am a big proponent of fewer rather than more reps, the reason being that you want to train more of your fast twitch fiber muscles. These are the muscles that you use mainly during short and fast movements. The golf swing happens to be a very short and mostly fast movement; from the static address position to the finish of the swing it usually takes no more than four to eight seconds.

The higher the number of reps, the more blood has to be transported to the muscles in order to supply energy, therefore the muscle will get bigger over time, which no "moving" athlete wants.

So, stay with the low range of reps and rather high weight and, no, you will not bulk up.

2. Sets:

The amount of sets will be noted with the workout programs. Many times you will see that some sets are done as super-sets, which means you will be doing back to back exercises of two opposite muscle groups without a break, e.g., doing a biceps exercise and a triceps exercise. As you work out the biceps, they will be fatigued for a short period of time. Working out the triceps right after that has the advantage that the fatigued biceps will not "work against" the triceps as much as an antagonist which may allow you to use more weight. Also, it will save you some time, as there is no break needed between the super-sets.

After three super-sets or between three sets of the same exercise, you should take about three minutes of rest, unless it is a low-intensity or learning exercise.

3. Weight:

I am a proponent of higher weight as well, as that fits in well with training the fast twitch fiber muscles and low reps. In order to get stronger, you need to overload your muscles which is best done with higher resistance versus higher repetitions as explained

earlier. That assumes that your body has been prepared and that you are performing the exercises perfectly.

Here is a good rule of thumb to find the right weight for an exercise. Let's say the program asks for eight reps with high weight for an exercise. Your seventh and eighth rep should be hard to do. If, after eight reps you are able to do two or three more reps, that means the weight you were using was too light and you should use a higher weight for the next set until you find it difficult to complete reps seven and eight.

4. Speed:

Speed has a very high impact on every movement you do — the higher the speed the more power you will produce. The right speed is also important when performing the exercises, especially during the eccentric (negative) phase of the exercise (whenever weight is moving towards the ground), as most strength will be built during that time as that puts the most strain on the muscle. More strain means that your body wants to adapt to the higher demand and therefore gives a signal to get stronger.

Some exercises, like a power clean, are to be performed at full speed during the concentric move (whenever the weight moves up) as you want to produce the highest power possible, as it is also during the concentric move that your body learns how to produce power.

Rhythm is another form of speed. For some exercises, especially the rotational ones you want to achieve about the same timing as in your swing with smooth and continuous transitions at every change of direction. Think of a pendulum, which is one of the most precise and efficient instruments there is — that's how you would like to move during the exercises that call for rhythm. This will give you a high carryover to your sport (think Annika or Ernie Els for rhythm)

Imagine someone suddenly pushing you during the golf swing or someone pushing against you with a slow and constant force, the latter would be much easier to control. That is the same if you compare a sudden acceleration to a constant (rhythmic) acceleration, the latter it is much easier to control.

5. Range of Motion:

Range of motion (ROM) plays an important part in good movement for leverage and power production. I prefer to call this ROM rather than flexibility. ROM is achieved through motion, while flexibility is often more of a static state. You can gain more flexibility by static stretching. For example, let's say I'm stretching my shoulders against a door frame. Statically, this gives me more flexibility but not necessarily more strength and control. The stabilizing muscles are not involved in that static stretching process and therefore don't get stronger or learn to stabilize. What you want to do is gain more ROM through the movement itself, meaning that, with most every exercise you do, you want to achieve full range of motion (without locking the joint). That's where you strengthen the stabilizing muscles as you gain ROM under load, which will give you more control but also greater protection for the joints.

Good ROM is also essential to take advantage of elastic strain energy — that's the energy you store in your muscles during a rhythmic move with a continuous transition at the change of direction, like transitioning from the back swing to the down swing. The longer and suppler your muscles are, the more energy you can build and release.

So, when performing an exercise, always make sure you go into full ROM without locking the joints — there should always be a slight bend in the joints, such as the elbows or knees. The difference between a straight joint and a locked joint may not appear much but makes a big difference in the amount of stress the ligaments and tendons have to contend with, as they are not made to stabilize. The muscles are responsible for that.

You should also not push the ROM to where you feel any discomfort or pain. Just be patient and your body will open up over time, if you keep asking it to do so.

The Principles

The Four Principles of Performing an Exercise

HERE ARE THE principles I teach and use every day with all of my students. They are the base of every exercise, and adhering to these principles will ensure that you will do the exercises that are right for you safely, as well as that you will benefit 100 percent from these workouts regardless of your sport.

The way I see it, the body must be trained as a complete chain from the toes up to the fingertips. A chain is only as strong as its weakest link, so there cannot be a weak link. This is true for any sport but is easy to understand if you look at the golf swing. You try your best to produce some movement in the club head in a certain direction with the intent to hit the ball just the way you like to. Basically you produce power through the activation of **all** the muscles in your body, that big interconnected system; not one muscle will be left out during the performance of a good swing.

The club acts as a tool as well as an extension of your limbs for better leverage.

Golfers spent much time, effort and money to select the right club. Each club consist of three basic parts: the grip, the shaft and the head. These three parts should always be well connected to each other, with no play between the grip and the shaft, or between the shaft and head, and the shaft must always be straight.

The same care has to be taken of your body. Considering how it is the sole source and control of power, it plays a big part of the success of your swing. To transfer that power to the ball in a controlled manner means it is critical to have that chain of body parts optimized in every way:

- A solid base from which to work (contact with the ground)

- Alignment of all body parts and spine angle

- Solid connection among all joints (core, muscles and connective tissue)

- Synchronization of all moving parts (nervous system)

- Uninterrupted transfer of power through the body (flow)

The question is, how do you learn all of this?

You know that your nervous system, which controls every move of your body, mostly learns by repetition and what your body does most it will remember best and therefore repeat when asked. For that reason you need to take your training seriously and concentrate on every move you do. No matter how easy you find an exercise to perform, it needs to be executed perfectly every time. I believe that the right training is divided into two parts, with 50 percent of your results being that you get mechanically stronger (muscles, connective tissue, flexibility etc.) and 50 percent improvement of the nervous system, knowing what muscle to fire at what time and at what intensity. The right firing order is very important as only then can your separate body parts move in a synchronized fashion to efficiently create, deliver and control power.

Picture a 100-piece orchestra, with every instrument played at the right time in the right sequence with the right volume. It sounds beautiful. But if just one instrument is out of sync or too loud, the perfect sound

cannot be achieved. It is the same with your swing. When every muscle is working at the right time in the right sequence with the right intensity, perfection is exhibited in generating that beautiful shot.

That is why it is so important that you do all these different exercises where you load up your body from all different angles and then learn how to produce power and control all the forces at the same time.

I am blessed to have worked with superb athletes like Annika, Darin Shapiro, Grant Hill, Will Asher, and Eddie Cheever, as well as some of the greatest from other sports, but I have also worked with high school and college players looking to achieve their full potential one day. The good thing is that I get to work with them one on one and therefore get their complete attention and concentration. That is what is needed to get the most out of their training.

I constantly remind them of their form while going through each motion to eliminate any "off" movement. The four principles I consistently reinforce as critical to every exercise are:

1. Feel the ground

2. Stay aligned

3. Abs in

4. Relax

These are the same four principles I

want you to use with every exercise you do. You have to understand they also have to work together just like all your body parts; they are integral to a successful movement. Every time you neglect one principle in any way you take away points from a 100 percent perfect move. Depending where you want to be, a few percentage points will make the difference between being good and being great.

Each of those principles has to be "activated" before every exercise, so before you start each repetition, activate each of them, and then perform that one repetition. So, when you plan on doing eight repetitions in a set of an exercise, think instead of doing it as eight times one repetition which means *you will activate all four principles eight times per set*. The more often you do it, the easier it is for your body to remember, and at some point they will come in place automatically, which will give you a high carryover to your sport.

You want to be able to deploy these principles automatically during your swing as well, therefore your body will listen and perform the way you like it to, rewarding you with that perfect shot.

Principle No. 1: <u>The Base</u> — Feel the ground

You know how important a good base is for any sport. Just try standing on some balance pads or on a steep slope in a bunker and instantly you wish for a better connection to the ground. When you move your limbs away from your body, you create a load and leverage that will affect your center of gravity. This load wants to pull you over. Just look at a crane to see how important the base is — the further away and the heavier the load, the stronger the base has to be. And, in the case of the swing, you need to add speed as yet another force.

Because you want to produce some power, you need the ground to push against in order to load up your muscles. If you are not well connected to the ground you miss out greatly on that effect. Also, the rotation during the swing creates yet another load that wants to move your body away from your base. Consider the force of the driver's head traveling at about 60 mph in the back swing and, in an instant you reverse the direction of that force as you turn to your down swing.

Off course balance has a great impact on your ability to hold your base. There are countless balance exercises available with tools (balance pads, gym ball, wobble boards etc.) or without (one leg exercises, on the toes, etc.).

I always prefer to perform exercises in a standing position whenever possible. For instance, if you do a seated row sitting on the floor or on a seated row machine with a bench, the sitting position will not help you to better your base. Your body will learn how to deal with that force in a sitting position and not standing. So, instead, do the row exercise standing up (called a Jockey Row), where your feet and legs will have to handle and distribute the load. Your nervous system will learn, and that way you have a better carryover to your "standing sport;" your body will remember. This explains, in addition to balance, engagement of the core, stabilizing muscles, and range of motion, why you should not use any exercise machines, as all those crucial elements are partially or completely neglected.

You need to realize how important the legs are in the swing as they are responsible for stabilization and production of power from the ground up, especially for women as they are generally weaker in the upper body and need to take advantage of their leg strength.

It is important that the knees remain slightly bent during any exercise for balance, stabilization, power production and the protection of your joints. As an experiment, stand up with your legs completely straight and try to jump without bending your knees. You will not go anywhere which tells you that, only if your knees are bent, can you use your leg muscles.

Get on your feet and move!

Here is how you do it. Imagine how you would like to stand if someone wanted to push you out of position: you should push your feet against the ground with your knees slightly bent — that's the position you need to be in for any standing exercise, no matter how easy or hard. With the feet about shoulder width apart, you want to feel your feet connected to the ground with the weight slightly distributed toward the front of each foot. This will require a little more effort than "just standing there." At the same time, you don't want to be all tight in your legs, which would take away from the ability to produce power; you want to have a bouncy feeling.

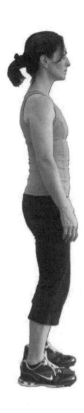
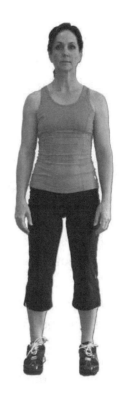

Here you see the right stance for working out: good alignment with your knees slightly bent and the weight slightly forward on your feet.

Principle No. 2:
The Axis — Stay aligned

Your axis, the spine angle, is your second setup point. As your body is centered around your spine, it is important to keep it this way while performing an exercise. The angle of your spine will influence balance and the production and transfer of power as well as directional control, i.e., of the dumbbell or the medicine ball (or the club). It is also important to keep the spine aligned to reduce stress, especially on the discs.

Think of a drive shaft in a car. Ideally you want the shaft to be straight. Any kink will produce extra stress on the connection points (joints), take away power and prevent it from running round and smoothly. Much energy gets wasted and the breaking point will be reached much earlier (in our case creating overuse or injury).

This is very similar to your spine. The power you produce through the use of your lower body, the midsection and upper body has to be transferred along the spine to your target point, like the dumbbell, medicine ball (or the club). Any deviation off that straight line will translate into loss of power. If your spine bends, your rotation cannot be as controlled and smooth, which means in the swing you never know where exactly your club head will end up. You will also have a hard time staying on your base as the forces on your body are greater and pull you laterally. Many times other parts of your body (e.g., the shoulders) try to compensate for the effect of a bad spine angle. This compensation often results in an overload of a certain joint or its connective tissue and overuse or injury will occur.

It is also important that your shoulders are kept square, parallel to the floor. If you dip or push down on one shoulder, the load on your spine will increase and the spine will have to bend.

Annika refers to the feeling in her swing of turning within a cylinder — there you cannot bend your spine. (See Annika Sorenstam, Golf Annika's Way.) This should be the same during any exercise. Your body will learn and transfer that new control to your swing.

For your exercises it is important to use a mirror whenever possible. Without being able to see the position of your body, you may not realize that your spine is actually bent or off axis — that may be your customary stance. Only by checking in the mirror will you be able to spot this. I have my players use one all the time. For me, as the trainer, I can see the spine angle from several directions through the mirrors and can correct them accordingly. A great help can be the point where two mirrors meet. Position yourself right in front of it and

line up your nose, belly button, and the center between your feet. Now you can see if you start moving your spine off the line. At home you can even take some masking tape and tape a "cylinder" the width of your shoulders onto the mirror. If you see yourself moving off the line and out of the cylinder, you want to find a way to correct it, or better yet, learn how to avoid it in the first place.

Good alignment in the spine is achieved by creating and holding a good base, by engaging your core muscles, maintaining good balance, keeping your shoulders square and staying aware of where your body parts are at any given time during the exercise. All this again has to be learned and constant checking in front of the mirror or by a trainer will help you control it.

Imagine a straight pole going through the center of your body. You cannot break that pole, so you need to avoid bending or sliding your hips or dipping your shoulders. That is also important during any rotation. It is very easy to bend your upper body or dip your shoulders during a rotational exercise. Again, think about the pole inside you and just rotate around it. You should always find your shoulders aligned above your hips and above the center of your stance.

I am a proponent of heavy weight exercises and eccentrics (after proper preparation). How should you lift a heavy dumbbell, for example, during a biceps curl where the load is trying to bend your spine to the side? Think again about the pole inside you, engage your core and with the help of your legs move down the pole and up in a pump like motion curling as you move upward through straightening your legs. This pump-like motion with the right timing will momentarily get you free of the weight so lifting it will be much easier. Some would call that cheating, I call it being efficient. The difference is that you do this in a safe manner with a straight spine and engaged core while distributing the load throughout the whole body.

The reality is that in most sports you have to deal with big loads and many times they come unexpectedly, so you must learn how to handle them through training. (Think of the driver travelling at over 70 mph. The centrifugal force wants to bend your spine as well). You want to be in charge of the dumbbell, the cable pull, the medicine ball, the club or any force that you create. Don't let it bend you out of shape!

On the left you can see a straight spine angle: the shoulders are aligned over the hips and the hips over the middle of the feet. On the right you see a misalignment as the shoulders are tilted. Watch yourself in the mirror!

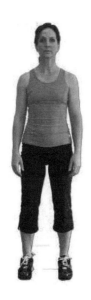
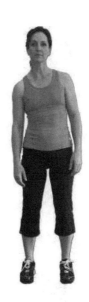

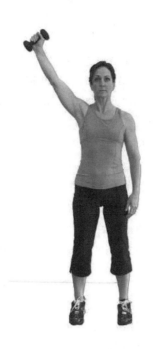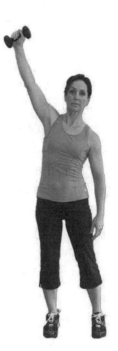

On the left you see good alignment. Even though the weight puts a side load on your body, you control the side load with the engagement of your abs. on the right you see "giving in" to the side load or compensating for weak abs and connection.

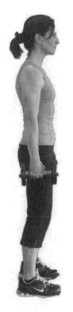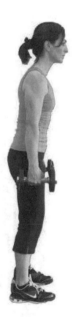

This is the side spine angle. On the left you see a neutral spine which is also aligned, shoulders over hips and ankles. On the right you see the upper body out of alignment. The shoulders are in front of the hips and ankles, which puts much more stress on your spine.

Principle No. 3: Abs in

The core — everywhere we look we find references made to the core. It is widely used by anybody having anything to do with fitness or golf. The core includes all the muscles between the ribcage and the pelvic floor, including the gluteus, and is responsible for connecting the lower body to the upper body and therefore transferring power, for rotation and stabilization of the hips and shoulders, as well as the protection of the spine.

Here I like to show you how I put the use of the core into application on an everyday basis through my training. Anybody I work with will tell you how often they get to hear from me: "abs in." I probably say it more than one hundred times a day.

The activation of the core will give you many benefits, including:

- connecting your upper and lower body to create one powerful unit

- transferring power from the bottom to the top of your body and vice versa

- creating stability

- creating rotational power

- protecting your spine

- keeping your spine angle straight

- compacting all the organs in your midsection and keeping them from wobbling around (and therefore not dispersing energy)

- defining the center of your body

- creating a nice, flat midsection (for that necessary beach look)

Many people have lost their ability to efficiently engage their core muscles or at least at the right time. This, combined with a very weak midsection, will often lead to lower back problems, no surprise today as many of us sit at a desk all day, stumble to the car to get home to find the couch before bedtime. This lack of engagement leads to many problems. Take, for example, when you bend over, rotate and reach to pick up something heavy out of the trunk of your car. The core is weak and not engaged, your spine is not protected and has to take care of the load, and that's when you can pull your back out, which can leave you lame for days.

You want to engage your core every time before you start moving any of the limbs to protect your spine from the created load and also to assure stability in your stance. To do this takes a lot of practice. It has to be done over and over again with every single move you take. Concentration and repetition is the key. You want to train your nervous system to be able to engage the core before initiating any movement of your limbs, and you want that engagement to become automatic by training it until it is embedded in your subconscious.

Now there are hundreds of core and abdominal exercises out there and they will get you a stronger mid-section but many of them have a poor carryover to the sport or everyday life, therefore, it is very important to use and train your core while performing your exercises, provided the exercises are free-moving and not restricted by machines.

Here is how I want you to engage your core. Standing in the upright position with your good base and straight spine, pull your belly button in and up. You should feel some pressure against your lower spine from the stomach wall pushing back; also, your gluteus should become engaged. In this position you might also feel that your ribcage has lifted somewhat and your breathing might be a little restricted. That is normal in the beginning as many of the core muscles are attached to the ribs. You want to learn how to disassociate your core from the upper body. Try to relax the upper and lower body adjacent to your midsection so they can move freely while your core is engaged. This will take some time and practice but once achieved will make a huge difference in your stability and strength.

There are two good ways to practice this. The first is to stand with your back against a wall with your heels, gluteus, shoulders and head resting against it. Now, place one hand behind the small of your back and draw your belly button in and up against the wall. Feel the pressure against your hand. In this position, learn to relax the rest of your body and try to breath relaxed as well. Hold for 20 to 30 seconds, then release and rest for 10 to 20 seconds. Repeat four or five times.

The second way is to get into the described position standing away from the wall. Again, the abs are pulled in and the rest of the body is relaxed. Now, rotate your upper body from one side to the other with your arms freely hanging. If you are relaxed, your arms should swing freely in front of you through the rotational forces while your core remains engaged through out. This "abs in" engagement needs to be started before any movement. I call the belly button the "start" button that has to be pushed in before the start of any move, no matter how simple.

Remember, you want to teach your nervous system to do it automatically every time so repetition is the key; you don't want to miss any opportunity to learn it.

For every exercise that has a change of direction, the core has to be re-engaged. For example, in a simple forward lunge, you set up your body and pull your abs in, then you step forward into the front lunge position. Just before the push with your front leg to get back to the starting position, you will re-engage your abs. This will keep you stable during the whole exercise and will help produce and transfer power from the upper and lower body to create a strong push back.

Again, your nervous system has to learn that re-engagement but, once learned, it can be used in the swing where, at the address of the ball, your core is set and just before the turnaround from the back swing to the down swing it will be reset again. That will give you stability and connection through the back swing and at the critical change of direction to the down swing.

Obviously we have to perfect this double engagement in order to be free to move and to be able to use it in the golf swing, but that's why we train and practice it with every movement we do in the gym. Within every rotational exercise this double engagement can be practiced in the same rhythm and timing as in your swing.

Another big advantage of engaging the core during the address of the ball is the ability to take the stress off your lower back muscles while supporting your upper body when leaning forward, which will prevent lower back pain and fatigue. You can test this yourself. While staying in your address position (with the upper body leaning forward), reach back with your hands and feel the muscles in your lower back just to the left and right of your spine (erector spinae). They are probably protruding out a bit and are tight. Now, engage your core while slightly tilting your hips underneath with your gluteus slightly engaged. When you reach back now, you will feel those muscles are now flatter and looser. That means that the load on your back muscles has been reduced and that you get more support from your core muscles, which are much better equipped to handle that stress. This is very evident when you do some prolonged putting practice — with the core engaged it will save you much lower back fatigue and pain.

That is also true when playing 18 holes, if your lower back muscles alone have to support your address position throughout the round you may feel towards the later part of the round that your swing is changing for the worse, your body is compensating for the fatigued lower back muscles. Don't let that happen and learn to use your core to support your posture.

Once you get very efficient and comfortable with the engagement and use of the core and you learn how to let your body work for you, you will be able to locate the center of your body, which is approximately one inch below your belly button. Think of rolling an egg and a ball next to each other on a flat surface. The egg's center is constantly changing so it will roll inconsistently, all over the place, where the round ball's center will stay consistent and rolls without any extra movement.

When your body learns to rotate around its center, all movement becomes much more efficient and almost effortless.

If you've ever struggled to open a mason or jelly jar, you probably instinctively held the jar close to your stomach, tightened your abs and only then tried to turn off the lid. That's using your core correctly, close to the center of your body.

Good core strength, but even more important knowing how to put the core into application during the swing, can lead to tremendous results. When I started to work with Karen Stupples in 2003, I realized that she was very strong in the lower and upper body but the connection was missing. I taught her how to use the core within her already very athletic swing, and she began driving the ball an extra 25 yards after only four weeks of training. That is the power of the core.

Annika is another example of this. Her swing has been very dependent on her ability to use the core to perfection, easy to see in cohesiveness of the whole body in her swing. During her pregnancy and the months following, her driving distance declined progressively even though her technique was still intact. The separation of the abdominal wall during pregnancy had weakened her core and compromised her connection and power transfer between the lower and upper bodies.

Here are some of the best exercises to practice this "abs in" move.

Supine Abs In. This may be the easiest way to learn how to engage your abs. As you lie relaxed flat on the floor, you will feel that there is some space between the small of your back and the floor. Try to close that space by engaging the abs through drawing your belly button to the floor and tilting your hips toward your upper body. When done right, you will feel that your gluteus will also engage. While holding this position you want to learn to relax the rest of your body — your chest, shoulders, arms, legs and also your breathing. This engaging of the abs and simultaneous relaxing of the rest of the body is not easy but can be practiced with easy exercises like this, holding for 20 to 30 seconds, and then releasing. Repeat 3 to 5 times.

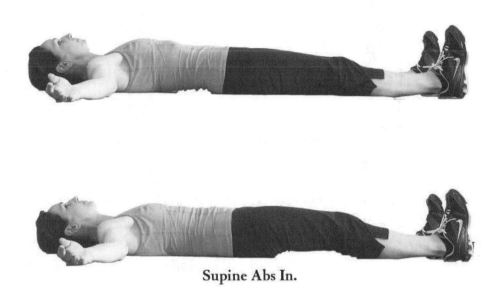

Supine Abs In.

Abs In Against The Wall. This is a great way to learn to engage the abs in the standing position. Keep your heels, gluteus, upper back and head against a wall, draw your abs toward the wall to close the gap between the small of your back and the wall, then slightly tilt your hips up and engage the gluteus. Here again, try to relax the rest of your body as well as your breathing, hold for 20 to 30 seconds, release and repeat 3 to 5 times more.

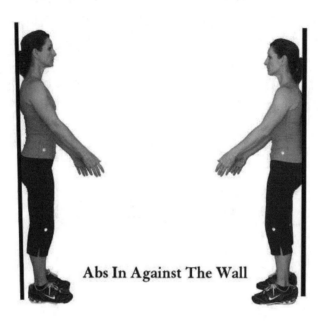

Abs In Against The Wall

Cat and Camel. This is another easy way to learn to engage the abs and tilt the hips. **# 1** is the neutral position with light abs and gluteus engagement and neutral hip tilt. Here in **# 2** the camel position the abs are not engaged, the tension of the erector spinae puts the hips into a negative tilt and the spine in a reverse C. Here in **# 3**, the cat position the hips are tilted to its maximum flexion with the abs engaged.

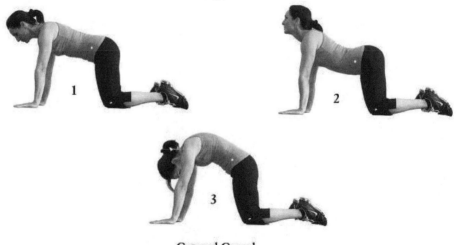

Cat and Camel

Abs In Standing. Abs In Standing. **#1** is a neutral, unengaged stance. **#2** is "abs in" stance with a light hip tilt and engagement of the gluteus – that's the right amount of hip tilt. Whereas, in picture **#3**, you can see that the hips are tilted too much, the lower back is too round, which in turn will put extra stress on the spine.

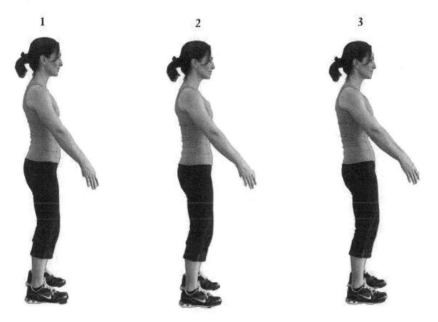

Abs In Standing

These principles of the correct use of the core have been confirmed by my good friend Dr. Christian Haid, a physicist and biomechanic at the University of Innsbruck, Austria. Christian received the prestigious Volvo Award from his research on the function and stress of the spinal discs. He is now a consultant to the Annika Academy for the development of the "Healthy Back for Golfers" program. Dr. Haid explains the importance of engaging the abs during the swing (as well as during all other physical activities). The right preloading of the core muscles will set the discs of the spine into a more neutral position between the vertebrae's and also strengthens the outer wall of the discs (Anulus fibrosus) which therefore can handle the stress of the swing much better.

We are fortunate to have Dr. Haid as our consultant, with his background in physics and bio mechanics he can proof (mathematically and through the laws of physics) many of the principles of a efficient, healthy and successful swing that we teach here at the Academy.

Following is an explanation in his own words about the use of the abs in the swing.

The function of the abs during the golf swing

By Dr. Christian Haid

THE ACCUMULATION OF all the core muscles connects the hips and pelvic floor to the upper trunk (chest, upper back), they are arranged in several layers running in different directions.

The core enables movement between the hip and the shoulder girdle as well as the bending of our upper body in different direction.

When you engage the abdominal muscles and at the same time your lower back muscles (antagonist's) with equivalent force there will be no movement which means you are bracing your spine through pre tension of the surrounding muscles. This is an important function to first protect the spine as well as improving the efficiency for movement.

Looking at **protecting the spine** the pre tensioned abdominals (abs in) will put your spine into a neutral position, therefore the vertebrae's are in a more favorable position (parallel) to transfer forces. The pressure on the (healthy) disc's is slightly increased through this pre tensioning which in turn will also increase the tension in the outer layers of the disc (annulus fibrosus) and therefore also increases stability throughout the spine. In this state the core muscles as well as the spine can work together to control and eliminate any unwanted forward or side bending. Also the amount of rotation is also better controlled (and slightly restricted) which means that the brunt of the rotational forces are handled by the surrounding muscles and not by the ligaments (due to better leverage of the muscles vs. the ligaments), reducing the stress on the surrounding joints.

In this state the spine is best equipped to handle the stresses of the swing (or any other rotational and lifting activity).

Looking at **movement efficiency** in the swing the pre tensioning of the abs (as well as all other torso muscles like the lats) will help you increase power. These muscles act like springs designed to work together. When you create some outside forces like lifting the club the pre tensioned muscles will be stretched, at the same time the muscles that run in the opposite direction will loose some tension which increases muscular strength without any activation, this happens automatically. Now additionally these pre tensioned "springs" (muscles) can be activated by concentrically pulling them together and therefore increasing the power optimally. In the swing this can be most efficient just before and during the down swing.

This pre tensioning also helps with a smooth and continuous strength increase which is important for a smooth and continuous acceleration.

During the swing the effective weight of the club increases, the faster the clubs speed the higher the centrifugal forces, the weight of the club can be many fold. Here too the pre tensioning of the abdominals (and subsequently the back muscles) will help compensate for the increase in the clubs weight (which wants to pull you forward and down) and maintain the desired spine angle.

In this picture you see Charlotta Sorenstam in her back swing position. At the end of the back swing rotation imagine that your muscles are "loaded" (eccentrically stretched) very similar to the rubber band you see here. This eccentric load stores energy which you want to use in your down swing. As explained earlier you want to make sure you reengage your abs just before the down swing to take advantage of the stored energy, that will create a good "snap" to accelerate the club. If you fail to do so that energy will dissipate into different body parts which in turn creates unwanted movement which will have to be stabilized. You see me getting ready to cut the stretched rubber band which would lead to the upper part of the band snapping up and the lower part snapping down, the energy is then gone. This also requires that you don't stop at the end of your back swing, create a continues and gradual transition as stopping would again dissipate the stored energy.

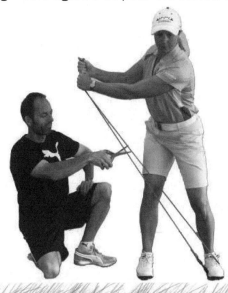

Principle No. 4: <u>Relax</u> — The Power of letting go

Power Flow is a term I came up with for this principle and I found it to be very fitting. When you lift an object or overcome resistance, like from the cable pull, you want to imagine that the forces that create that movement are flowing through your body (a physicist will call those "impulses" which travel through your body much like electricity).

This is very important. These forces need to be able to flow freely in order to transfer the energy efficiently to where it is most needed. In the case of weightlifting, it may be the dumbbell that's moving, or, in case of a golfer, the energy should flow through your body to the shaft and club head to be transferred to the ball. If you block or restrict that flow, much of the created energy will be wasted, and get's "stuck" inside your body, which translates into poor efficiency.

You've no doubt had that experience before. Imagine your best drive — it's long and straight, just perfect. Now, if I would ask you right after that swing, "What did you feel?" could you tell me? Most people say they did not feel anything, it was easy, effortless. That is what happens when all the energy you created was directed to precisely the right place (it was able to flow freely). You used the right muscles at the right time in the right sequence with the right volume. This is the same feeling that you want to create in the gym when you work out. Let your body move freely, relax your grip, be soft in your legs. The only part of your body that should consciously be engaged is your core. (Note: I'm saying engaged, not tensed.)

Think of how easy it is for you to walk — you don't even feel your weight. You learned to walk very early in life and it is very natural to you; you relax and let your body move freely. Now, try tightening up any part of your body like a toe or your fist and start walking. Not long and you will start feeling your weight, other body parts have to start to compensate, some joints will start to hurt at some point, much of the energy created cannot flow and, thus, puts extra stress on your system.

Your body wants to move in the path of least resistance, if you will let it. Too often you make things more complicated than necessary, which will only get in your way and cause more stress as the energy created has to go somewhere but you're not letting it flow along that path of least resistance.

What gets in the way of the flow are the simultaneously activated agonistic and antagonistic (opposite) muscles. For example, if you tighten your biceps and triceps at the same time with the same intensity, your forearm will not move even though you are expending a lot of energy. Release the biceps and your forearm will move away from your body, the triceps now can create movement free of restriction, as the biceps is not pulling against it anymore. The opposite is true as well, when you release the triceps.

Again, you want to learn to let forces flow unimpeded through your body. Don't restrict. Relax and you will become very efficient. That does not mean that you go easy in the gym! I want you to lift heavy weights at times, but try to make it look and feel as easy as possible.

This throws a lot of bodybuilding techniques out the window. When in the gym, you will still hear about "squeezing" or "isolating" your muscles, and that is fine if all you want to do is to bulk up and have no interest in efficient movement, but if you want to be able to move efficiently, (and I know you want to, because that's why you

got this book) then stay away from that technique. Remember the story I told you about the bodybuilding sky diver.

I currently work with Shannon Aubert, a member of the French Junior National Team. In 2010, at the age of 14 she weighed in at 85 pounds, and she drove the ball 240 yards. I call that being efficient. The energy she creates goes to the right places without restriction, and that's what you should be striving for.

The cable concentration curl is a great example to feel the "power flow." Your arms are completely relaxed with a loose grip. Now imagine the forces flowing from the end of the cable through your fingers, hands, forearms, upper arms, shoulders, chest and back into the core. When curling, maintain that flow by staying relaxed and getting help from your core by engaging the abs. Curl the arm and don't tighten any body part. Feel how your abs help you here. Just

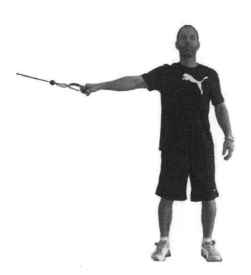
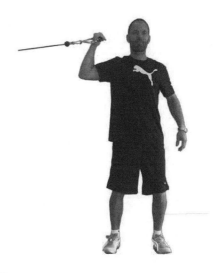

imagine you want to let water run from the cable to your midsection through that chain of body parts. If you "squeeze" any of these parts, the flow of water will be restricted.

This is a great way to feel the "letting go" and "swing effect". With a light weight loose in your hand feel like your arm is just a pendulum hinged by the shoulder and let the weight swing from side to side. It is amazing how effortless it can be to create some speed in the moving dumbbell. As soon as you tighten any part of your body you will feel that the easy pendulum effect is gone. Try to get that feeling during your swing, you will see your distance increase immediately.

Granted it is harder during the swing as both arms are connected at the grip of the club.Therefore the shoulders are connected through your arms, this connection turns your two single shoulders from a "ball joint" into a "hinge joint" and more opposite (antagonistic) muscles can work against you...but practice will make you perfect.

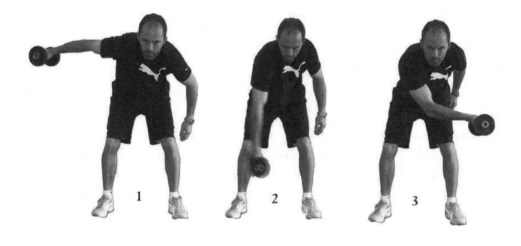

Part 3

Back Pain

Now I DON'T have any solid statistics on this but from my experience I would say that about 30% of golfers experience some kind of lower back pain, may it be of muscular or structural nature.

Realize that the motion of the swing: forward lean, rotation, dipping, acceleration and deceleration can put tremendous forces on the spine and its surrounding tissues like the ligaments and discs of the spine. These forces are especially high if the surrounding and supporting muscles are weak, not engaged or both.

Some of these forces are inevitable but with the biomechanically right movement pattern, engagement of the supporting and stabilizing muscles as well as gradual and continuous acceleration and deceleration they can be minimized.

Sometimes players think that a "healthy" swing can't be a good swing, naturally I will tell you that Annika's swing had both elements in spades, healthy **and** good.

Following are the most important principles to put in place in order to minimize the stress on your body during the swing. And theses principles will not only safe your back but all the other joints as well like the shoulders, elbows and knees.

1. **Muscular Pre Tension**
   As explained by Dr. Haid in the abs section of this book, pre tensing the right muscles at the right time will protect your joints by minimizing the load on the ligaments and by increasing the efficiency.

2. **Biomechanical Geometry**
   Keeping a biomechanically correct geometry is important to minimize the forces on the joints. This is just simple physics; ideally all the limbs should be aligned with the torso (and therefore spine) so the forces don't have to travel through angles. The spine angles should be maintained throughout the rotation without any side (i.e. hip slide) or forward bending (i.e. dipping).

3. **Avoid maximum Range of Motion**

Extending or rotating into the full range of motion in the swing will lead to extra stress on the ligaments of the spine and joints, avoid this by using your muscles to stabilize and protect the joints.

4. **Gradual Acceleration and Deceleration**

As explained in the previous chapters learn to have gradual and linear changes of speed in order to avoid speed spikes which induce instability and therefore extra stress on the joints.

5. **Let it Flow – Release**

As explained in the Power Flow section, let the forces flow through your body which also means that you will not "tighten up" (let go of the antagonistic muscles), release the energy created to the intended target like the club head and subsequently the ball. Not releasing will keep the energy in your body and again adds stress to the spine and the joints.

6. **Sufficient Warm-up**

As explained in the warm-up section, your muscles need to be warmed up sufficiently to be able to react and protect the ligaments of the spine and joints

7. **The right club length**

This is an often over looked problem. If the club is too short you will inevitably have to bend forward in order to still hit the ball (and our brain will almost always make sure you will always hit the ball no matter the physical consequences). This forward bending during the highest upper body speed in the down swing puts tremendous forces on the spine and its ligaments. To avoid this get fitted for the right club length, rather go longer then too short.

WEIGHT TRAINING FOR GOLF

(pictures courtesy of Dr. Christian Haid)

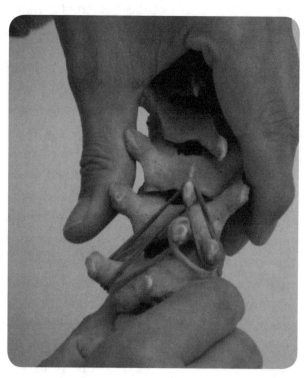

Picture # 1: in this make up of the spine you see muscles (rubber bands) attached to the facets of the vertebrae's, as you rotate your spine the muscles in direction of the rotation get stretched (or pre-loaded) as the opposite muscles loosen up.

PRESSURE DISTRIBUTION IN THE DISC

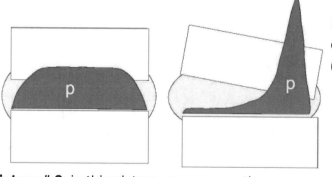

High pressure in the outer parts of the disc (anulus fibrosus)

Picture # 2: in this picture you can see the pressure distribution on the disc of the spine, on the left the vertebrae are parallel to each other and the pressure on the disc is evenly distributed. On the right the vertebrae are tilted to each other which leads to pressure peaks on the disc. That's why any unnecessary bending of the spine should be avoided. Engaging the core as described will also help to keep the vertebrae more parallel to each other.

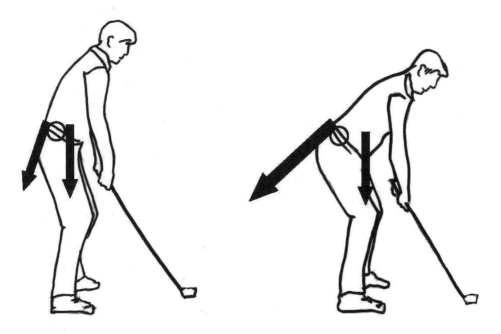

Picture # 3: here you can see the comparison between a more upright stance vs. a more bent over stance, the more we bend over the higher the muscular forces (see force vectors) on the back i.e. due to a too short of a club.

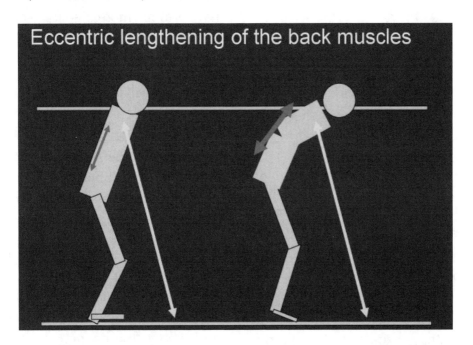

Eccentric lengthening of the back muscles

Picture # 4: here you can see how the muscular forces in the back increase dramatically (see force vectors) if you increase your bend of the spine during the swing at high speed (here due to rising up on your toes during the down swing). Keep your spine angle the same throughout the swing.

Are You Still Doing Cardio?

WALK INTO ANY gym and the first thing you see is people straddling treadmills, elliptical machines or bikes for 45 minutes or more, trying to burn calories and improve their aerobic fitness (all while watching their favorite show on TV).

I see and hear this all the time, especially from the ladies, this notion that you need a good long sweat in order to get a good workout and burn lots of calories. I suspect that some people are actually addicted to that type of cardio workout.

It is not easy to convince people why they should steer away from the typical low- to moderate-intensity continuous training (cardio) and instead do sprint interval training (also known as HIIT, or burst training). After all, we have been conditioned by many alleged fitness experts and health professionals to believe we need make several 30 to 45 minutes sessions of cardiovascular training every week to stay fit, healthy and burn fat.

I'm not saying that doing slow and long cardio is all bad and that you should never do it. I know many people feel that they get a great deal of mental stress relief and I can't argue with that, but from a purely physical stand point it is not at all efficient and may harm you more then it will do you good.

As I am not a physician or a biophysicist, I will leave the more technical scientific explanations of this subject to Dr. Izumi Tabata, whose research is readily available online as well as the publication and collected research by Mark J. Smith, PhD (www.x-iser.com).

Slow cardio is very time intensive (the number one reason people skip their workouts), only works on your aerobic fitness (and that fairly inefficiently), burns only moderate calories during the activity yet has no impact on your metabolism (the decline of our metabolism is what many of us are fighting as we get older), and stresses your joints due to repetitive impact (especially running). It also increases inflammation.

Now, here is a solution for you. It's called HIIT (high intensity interval training) or burst training. *And it only takes about four to eight minutes, three times per week!* Yes, you read that right. Understand that more is not better in this case; it's the intensity, not the duration that best affects the adaptation to exercise and that makes the difference.

It works both your aerobic and anaerobic systems at the same time and is very effective for fat loss. It will also raise your metabolism for several hours afterward, build "fast muscles" and reduce impact to your joints and even help reduce inflammation. HIIT training can burn the same calories as slow cardio in one-fifteenth (less than seven percent) of the time! That means that just four minutes of HIIT equals an entire hour of slow cardio! Slow cardio produces a lot of stress hormones (cortisol) while sprint training stimulates growth hormone. Ever compared the physique of a sprinter to that of a marathon runner? Which would you prefer?

There are different ways to implement HIIT training. It can be done on equipment, like a treadmill (remember, now you're pushing the belt with the machine turned off), stationary bike, upper body ergo meter, a X-iser or jump rope. It can also be done with no equipment at all, like sprinting (athletes only), running in place with high knees, running up a flight of stairs, up a hill or with full body calisthenics like Turkish getups or push-ups to jumps.

I recommend starting with four-minute workouts (adding two to three minutes of warm-up beforehand) with a sprint to rest ratio of 1:3, say, a 10-second sprint (fast pace) with a 30-second rest (slow pace). As you start to feel more comfortable with this, you should work your way down to a ratio of 1:1, such as a 20-second sprint followed by a 20-second rest. The maximum total time you would want to exert yourself here is six to eight minutes.

Remember that the sprints should be high intensity, which is of course relative to your fitness level. On a scale of 1 to 10, your effort during the sprints should be a 10! If you feel that your sprints are losing intensity that means the sprint time is too long or the rest time too short, adjust accordingly.

With my athletes, I never do any slow cardio; it would take up too much of their time. Every minute we have to train, I want to make sure that they get a 100 percent return of their time invested. With slow cardio, the rate of return is just not high enough, plus, I always felt that if you do a lot of "slow" training, it will make you slow and that is not what you want in any sport. Remember that speed is a big component of power in the swing.

Another factor to consider is the ability to learn to turn your system on and off. During the sprint time, you turn everything on full power, 100 percent, and during the rest period everything needs to be turned off in order to recuperate and get ready for the next sprint. That is very similar to playing golf. When you are hitting the ball you want your whole system to be turned on, while between the shots you want to turn everything off and preserve energy. After all, it would be very hard to stay on full power for the four to five hours that a typical round will take. You would run out of energy.

Annika likes the jump rope for HIIT, as it's really great for the coordination but it also teaches you to relax; otherwise you would trip over the rope constantly. She would do 20 seconds slowly than 20 seconds at full speed followed by 20 seconds slowly, etc., for four to six minutes, all that three or four times a week. It served her very well over the years, she had plenty of endurance during her tournaments (like the 2006 US Open she won after an extra playoff round).

By the way, I use the same training method for my son's soccer team and other athletes who are competing in

high aerobic sports, and it works very well.

You will be surprised how fast your body will adapt to the new and positive exercise stress. Your energy level will increase, performance will improve, metabolism will pick up, you will save time and wear on your joints, and, most of all, it's a lot more fun!

Here some examples:

1. Upper body ergo meter. This is one of my favorites for HIIT training. It's also great for the arms and shoulders. Make sure you stand up (slide the chair back if equipped with one) and keep your knees bent, relax your grip and get help from your whole body. Alternate going forward and backward, starting with a 30-second slow to 10-second sprint ratio and work up to a 20-second slow to 20-second sprint when strong enough.

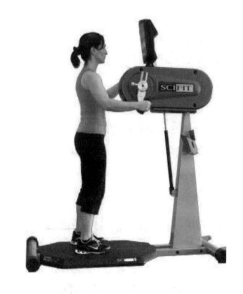

2. Pushing the treadmill. This is the real deal. It will train your whole body without much impact, and it's great to strengthen the legs and gluteus. You will learn to "drive" and not jump. Turn the motor off completely (switch in the back) or unplug the machine, hold onto the handrail without locking your arms and push the belt back. It's OK if you lean forward somewhat. Walk for 30 seconds, then sprint for five to ten seconds to start with. When you start getting stronger, you can work yourself up to a ratio of 20 seconds walking to 10 seconds sprinting.

3. Running in Place. This is an easy one to do almost anywhere. You will be amazed how much you will use your abs during the high knees. Do some light jogging in place for the slow portion and sprint to full speed with high knees and arms pumping. Start with 30 seconds of slow jogging, followed by 10 seconds of high knee sprinting, when getting stronger you can get to 20 seconds of slow running to 20 seconds of sprinting.

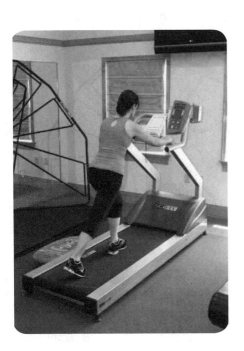

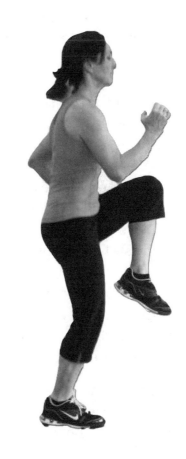

KAI FUSSER

Recuperation and Stretching

DEPENDING ON YOUR goals, you want to train your body as hard as possible in order to achieve the necessary gains. That puts a certain amount of stress on your body, physically and mentally. For the golf pros, you work out with high intensity for one hour in the morning followed by practice for several hours and play some holes as well; that's a little bit of a Catch-22 situation. That's where recuperation and rest play such a big role. If you don't help your body along with that, it will shut down at some point, injuries will appear, you may experience that fatigue, speed, power, coordination and more will be compromised.

Sleep may be the biggest factor in recuperation. Research shows that a minimum of 9 hours of sleep each night is necessary for your body to be able to repair the mind and body from the stresses of the day. I can tell you that all my high performance athletes are really good sleepers. They have the ability to turn a switch and go to sleep almost on the spot, and stay that way for 10 hours! That's certainly a gift and you should try your best to learn that. Only during sleep can your body and mind repair.

Proper nutrition is another important factor for recuperation. Food is the only source of energy for our body and we cannot repair our muscles, soft tissue, cells, etc., without it. In the nutritional section of this book you will learn what to eat and when for optimum recovery.

A hands-on approach to recuperation can include stretching, either manual stretching by lengthening your muscles through a pulling action, or by using a foam roller which is basically a self-controlled form of a deep tissue massage. As I mentioned in the warm-up section of this book, there is no real and clear evidence that stretching will help prevent injury or aid in recuperation, but I have to say that, through personal experience and anecdotal evidence, stretching can have a positive effect on recuperation if it is done right. Much of the success will also have to do with what you feel as our beliefs play a role in the perceived outcome as well.

There are several rules that you should follow in order to stretch safely.

You need to make sure that your body is completely warmed up before stretching, otherwise the muscles will not let go and the end result will be a pull on the ligaments and tendons, which could lead to injury. That's one of the reasons why many people get into trouble by stretching before hitting balls right out of the car, without any warm-up. That's why I recommend the warm-up to consist of controlled dynamic movements with a full range of motion. So make sure to have the muscles warmed up before stretching them and that also includes being in a warm environment, not standing on the range in 45-degree temperatures with 20-mph winds. It is also important that the muscles to be stretched are relaxed, after all you are trying to lengthen the muscle and that is not possible if they pull against your stretch. Equally so if you are trying to stretch a muscle that is already busy stabilizing your body, such as performing a standing hamstring stretch where the hamstring is engaged keeping you from falling over.

The duration of the stretch is important as well. It takes time for the muscles to "let go." Don't rush it; take at least 45 seconds for each stretch. I think that stretching can also have a mental relaxation component, so relax everything and take your time.

The force applied during the stretch should be minimal and gradual, otherwise injury can occur. Do not bounce or rapidly pull to stretch or you will pull your muscle and that's what you wanted to prevent in the first place. I often hear athletes say (especially in the soccer world): "I pulled my hamstring and I need to stretch it out." No! You just pulled the muscle or ligament, why would you keep pulling on it even more? Let it rest.

You also have to be careful after a really hard workout not to stretch the affected muscles too early. Through the overload stress, they are prone to injury if stretched too early. Wait at least 45 minutes and then start with a light stretch.

I do like the use of rubber bands a lot more than stretching against a solid object like a bar or pole. With the band it is much easier to just let your weight sink into it (as it is stretchy vs. rigid) with a loose and relaxed grip. It also gives you many different angles to get into to find the right spot to be stretched.

The same rules apply to the foam roller. Understand that the foam roller can apply enormous pressure on your muscles as it spreads the muscle fibers apart with high pressure, depending on how much weight you apply. That is, you can roll the hamstrings together at the same time with the weight of the legs distributed to both hamstrings equally or you fold one hamstring on top of the other and now one has to bear the weight of both of them; the pressure is now double. Also, start easy when you roll areas where there is not much muscle tissue between the skin and the bone, like the shins, as you could bruise the muscle and the skin easily if overdone and the pain the next day will give you a good reminder.

The stretches I show in this book I find to be some of the most effective ones. There are many more that you can do, just make sure you consider the rules as shown. Make sure it feels good and use it as a constructive down time.

The Mind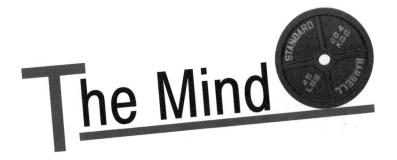

YOU MAY WONDER why I have included a chapter on the mind in a workout book. Well, that is very easy to answer. Without your mind you can't plan ahead, you would live only in the present (the present supposedly is about 3 seconds long; anything before or after that exists in the past or future) which would mean that you can't set goals or prepare. Every action you take every day, may it be as simple as brushing your teeth in the morning, requires goal setting and forethought — you see yourself do it and then you act on it. That basic but very important concept needs to be understood and then put into planned application to help you reach your goal.

I am passing this chapter on to Gregg Cochlan, a facilitator for The Pacific Institute (TPI) out of Seattle, WA, founded and led by Lou Tice, a master of cognitive psychology teaching. My friend, Bob Ferguson, also a facilitator, introduced me to Lou Tice and TPI (which led me to become a facilitator myself). Bob and Gregg both held the TPI psychology courses at the ANNIKA Academy for our entire team but also for my athletes like Annika, Anna Nordqvist and Graeme McDowell.

I use these concepts on an everyday basis, it's part of my coaching in the gym, for my personal/family life as well as with all my students. Staying positive, setting goals, thinking forward, seeing the good, and positive self-talk are all things that you should incorporate every day, as it will put you on the straightest path to where you want to be. All good things start in the mind. Learn how to use it.

I encourage you to read up on some of the excellent material available on this topic, as it can make a huge impact on your life and the ones you touch. You will find some resources in the recommended reading and resource section of this book.

KAI FUSSER

Managing your Mind - The Competitive Advantage

by Gregg Cochlan

IN GOLF, HAVE you ever thought about a course you are going to play and visualized the holes? As you get to some of these holes in your mind, you might see a positive outcome — a par or birdie — but for some other holes, you see images of triple bogeys. What thoughts go through a PGA player's mind when they think of number twelve at Augusta or the island green at The Players? Are they thinking about a positive outcome or are there flashes of the negative? For amateurs, if we ever got to play these holes, would some of you pull out an old ball to play them?

A term in cognitive psychology that may be useful for you at this point is "forethought." Forethought is the ability for human beings to think into the future, to actually think creatively and positively about future events. The good news on this is it allows us to set and build goal images about things we want to achieve. It can be as simple as daydreaming or as complex as strategic planning. It allows us to visualize what we want — in the future. So, many people look forward into the future with positive expectancy, with a "I can hardly wait" expectancy. They are looking forward and thinking this is going to be great. This is what I train for; I love this type of pressure. This is the thought process that high performance people recognize and use regularly. They look forward with positive expectancy. They visualize success. They expect to win. They practice in their mind before the event. They "teach" themselves a positive outcome.

The flip side of this human functioning is negative forethought, which is usually not good. People look forward, but they look forward with a negative expectancy. They spend time visualizing what may or will go wrong. They worry. Worry is considered to be negative goal setting. You are visualizing what you <u>don't</u> want to happen.

It is fun when you start to play around with this concept of forethought and apply it to training. Are there some exercises you look forward to and some you want to creatively avoid?

Here are a couple of strategies that may help you manage your mind in difficult environments. One is to be aware of forethought and become very aware of what you are visualizing. If your mind wanders into thinking about what could go wrong, STOP! Instead, START putting in replacement pictures of you successfully playing the shot or doing the drill flawlessly. Second, become aware of your conversation as you are visualizing. If it's positive, deepen it. If it's negative, stop it. Find a trigger thought that you can replace it with. If your thought may be: I miss three-foot putts, replace it with: I always make them, center of the cup, and visualize the sound of the ball dropping in. Managing your mind is managing your thoughts, controlling your forethought.

In cognitive psychology, we have a formula: B (behavior) = H (heredity) + E (environment) + HA (human agency).

It is used to describe how your thinking affects your performance. Your **B**ehavior is the result of your **H**eredity & **E**nvironment & **H**uman **A**gency (Thinking). This is important because, while you have very little control over your heredity and only limited control over your environment, you have total control over your thinking.

This is an important fact, because if you can control your thinking, environment can play less of a role in affecting your performance. In life or in sport or in fitness, those individuals who become skilled at managing their minds or controlling their thinking clearly have a competitive advantage. It is why in the last seconds of a basketball game, Michael Jordan always wanted the ball, or in hockey's Stanley Cup final, Wayne Gretzky always wanted the puck. Many players would let the environment or a tension of the game get in the way of their great performance when, in fact, they want this pressure — this is why they play the game.

Great players don't let the environment negatively affect their performance. It is mind over environment, and, in some cases, even mind over heredity.

Now that's a competitive advantage!

Now that you have the key idea, let's talk about practice. Like a workout, it takes practice to get the exercise done properly. Throughout this book, Kai provides you with proper drills and techniques, which will take practice to nail down and perform correctly. In golf, hitting a three-iron "pure" takes practice. Managing your mind is the same; it takes practice. Practice managing your forethought, practice putting in positive replacement pictures, and practice placing positive expectancy into your game.

You can control your environment and your performance by managing your mind.

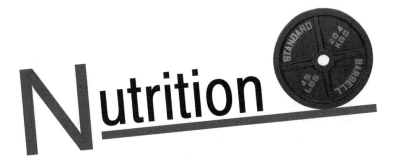Nutrition

How CAN I cover a topic this important in just one chapter? There are probably several thousands of books on nutrition and diets, some good, some bad, and some downright ugly. It's a huge industry now and everyone sooner or later will have some dealings with it.

Many times nutrition is portrayed as a very complex and complicated matter. I don't think it has to be that way. Even though there is much to be learned, common sense should still prevail.

Of course, nutrition is very important for athletic performance, just like it is for everyday life and long-term health, even for our emotional health. I always like to give some simple explanations and then you can draw your own conclusions.

1. What goes from your hand into your mouth is your decision and your decision alone (unless your mother still feeds you); and

2. What you eat today is what your body will consist of in about one year from now (our body rebuilds itself in about one year).

See? That's pretty simple.

Realize that our body is nothing more than a chemical reaction that goes on 24 hours a day, seven days a week. There are certain ingredients in certain ratios that need to be right in order for our system to function at 100 percent the way it was designed. If you mess with these chemicals and ratios by missing certain ingredients or by introducing ingredients into your system that don't belong, then something will have to give. It could be loss of energy at first, or some outer appearance changes (to put it nicely), inflammation, dysfunction of your system, cancer, etc.

It's the cumulative effect that creates problems down the road, for some earlier, for some later. In your teens and twenties, your body is more resilient and what you consume then does not seem so critical (at least it does not show up yet), but as you get older your body gets less forgiving. You also know now that your body renews itself every year or so, that's good news as it will never be too late to make good changes and the results will show and be felt.

Your body was designed a very long time ago and only in the last 50 years or so have we introduced all these new chemicals which the body can't recognize or process. Maybe in a 100 or more years from now, people will adapt to it, but as of right now you have to adjust and deal with them.

I suggest you learn as much as you can about nutrition and then apply your knowledge to your everyday live without getting too paranoid about it. I like the 80/20 rule here: 80 percent good and 20 percent just OK. If you have built a good base from wholesome and clean food, then it's OK to have something not so good, that occasional moderate ice cream or chocolate can be tolerated without repercussion. If you splurge, stay away from the "artificial" sin full of chemicals — get the real deal, like full fat full sugar ice cream and get it over with. You will do more harm to your body by consuming the fat-free, sugar-free, colored, artificial look-alike ice cream. Those would be your typical junk foods.

I conducted an experiment about 13 years ago. On a road trip I bought a bacon cheeseburger from a well-known interstate fast food supplier. I left it in its wrapper — bun, meat patty, cheese and bacon — until I got home, then transferred it to a plastic container and never put it in the fridge. In those 13 years, this "thing" never went bad! No mold or any dis-

figuration. I have used it over the years whenever I do some nutritional seminars and showed it to the participants as shock therapy with great effect. (Sadly, a few months ago I came to my office at the Academy and the burger was missing from my desk. Later we found the empty plastic container that had been cleaned and left in the kitchen, so the cleaning crew must have thrown the 13-year-old burger out or they ate it. We never found out.)

Learn to read the food labels as they can be very deceiving. There are many catchphrases now like "fat-free," "sugar-free," "cholesterol-free," etc., if you see that on the label you have to ask yourself, how it can still taste like anything? The taste is created through added chemicals which only create havoc in your system Stay away from it! You can find some good websites that explain food labels and what they mean.

It also helps to write down what you are eating, to keep a diary of it. You would be surprised at what you learn when you do that. Just the act of writing it down creates some kind of self-accountability, plus, only then can you see how much protein, carbohydrates and fat you truly consume. You will see later in this chapter how much that matters. All my athletes provide me with that list periodically so we can see where their intake is and then we adjust accordingly.

Should you be calorie counting? Not necessarily. If you are eating very healthy, complete and wholesome food, your body will tell you when you are full. If you want to count calories I would go with the following formula, provided that you are an active person: calculate the amount of protein, carbohydrates and fat needed according to your desired body weight (see more about this later in this chapter) and multiply the protein and carbohydrate grams by 4 and the fat grams by 9 and you get your approximate caloric need.

Here is an example:

Body weight = 150 lbs

150 lbs x 0.8 = 120 g of protein

150 lbs x 2.5 = 375 g of carbohydrates

Total = 495 g x 4 = 1980 calories
(1g of protein or carbohydrates = 4 cal)

+ 10% for fat   = 198 calories
(= 22 g of fat, 1g of fat = 9 cal)

Total calories per day = 2,178

This is the formula that I use as a base for my athletes, we start there and then adjust accordingly if needed depending on the individual. Variations depend on how the energy level or recuperation is effected, or i.e. if there is a tournament week in a very hot climate some carbohydrates would have to be added.

I also suggest preparing as much as possible yourself, have the right foods at home, when you leave for the day bring healthy foods and snacks with you, and don't get caught hungry as the next thing that jumps your way is usually not the best choice.

Now, about supplements: I am a big proponent of supplementation *if* it is used right and has the right quality. In a perfect world, you might be OK without it but that is hardly the case anymore. There are many new and added stresses on our system today which warrant some offsetting. For my athletes it is critical as they want to perform at the highest level possible. At the same time they have the added stress from training, competing, travelling and more. They travel almost 40 weeks out of the year and you can imagine what the food choices are between airports, hotels and golf courses. That's when supplementation comes into play to fill the void and strengthen the immune system.

The question is how to navigate your way through the confusing and unregulated supplement market. There are literally hundreds of companies out there peddling their latest miracle concoction. I have seen some pretty scary stuff over the years as I am constantly approached to try out and recommend their products.

For me it is very critical what I recommend to my athletes, not only from a safety and effectiveness standpoint but also from the standpoint of drug testing, as all of them are periodically and randomly tested. I even have a waiver that my athletes have to sign, stating that if they use anything other than what I recommend, I take no responsibility.

Do not just go to any supplement store or company to buy a product without doing some thorough research on it. The supplement marketplace is poorly regulated and there are many products out on the free market that have ingredients that will show up as a banned substance!

The best way is to ask the manufacturer for their peer reviewed and published studies on their product, which you will see can be very hard to find.

I have used and recommended products from the Shaklee Corporation exclusively for the last 15 years, all my athletes are using them and we have had great success. I know their research and manufacturing process is impeccable and I trust them for safety and effectiveness.

You can find some great resources regarding Shaklee products, how I use them, nutritional tips and more on the www.FusserFitnessandNutrition.com website.

Here is a list of the main supplements that most of my athletes and I use:

1. **Recuperation:** a shake should consist of whey protein and carbohydrates at a ratio of about 1 part protein (about 20 to 30 grams) to 2.5 parts carbohydrates (about 50 to 75 grams). Drink within 20 minutes after a workout. Many of my players like to drink this type of shake at the turn of a round — it's easy to carry, gives you needed nutrients and is easy and quick to digest.

2. **Meal replacement:** a shake consisting of soy protein (intact, cold water processed, GMO-free, approximately 20 to 25 grams), carbohydrates (approximately 40 to 50 grams) and fiber (approximately 5 to 10 grams), or a bar with about the same ratios. Drink a shake instead of skipping meals or substituting a bad meal; add nutrition to meet your intake needs.

3. **Electrolyte replacement:** an electrolyte drink for use before and during prolonged physical activity over one hour (not your typical color-laced convenience store drink! You know which ones I am referring to)

4. **Vitamins:** a well-balanced and complete vitamin for immune and bodily functional system improvement. It should dissolve very quickly or your body will not be able to absorb it, beware of harmful fillers and binders.

5. **Fish oils and glucosamine:** to fight inflammation and promote joint health. Fish oils have to be of the highest quality as many brands are contaminated with heavy metals like mercury.

As I am not a nutritionist, I have asked my friend, Dr. Steve Chaney, to write some simple rules to healthy eating and explain the need for the right nutrients to support the higher demands due to physical training. Dr. Chaney has taught biochemistry and nutrition to medical students at the University of North Carolina for more than 30 years and is also a research specialist and author of more than 100 scholarly papers. He is also my go-to source to find and understand research papers and studies on nutrition.

Nutritional Support for Training and Playing

Dr. Stephen G. Chaney, PhD

Top 10 Tips for a Nutritious Diet to Support Both Health and Exercise

Every discussion of nutrition should start with a healthy diet, and that is just as true for sports nutrition as it is for any other kind of nutrition program. Here are my top 10 tips for a healthier diet.

#1: Eat a variety of foods from all of the five food groups that the USDA considers to be healthy. Without this, there is no way that we can be assured of receiving all the nutrients essential to good health. One of the major drawbacks of the fast food restaurants so popular in our society is the lack of variety in what they offer. The five healthy food groups are protein (meat, beans, eggs & nuts), dairy, fresh fruits, fresh vegetables, and whole grains. Unfortunately, most of the food we eat is from the sixth (unhealthy) food group—junk and convenience foods. These foods often supply us with so few nutrients that they cannot be considered a part of the basic five. For example, pizza theoretically provides foods from all five food groups, but if it is made from white flour, artificial tomato paste, and imitation cheese, it will, in fact, supply the body with very little of what it needs.

#2: Eat less fatty meats, especially red meat. Few of us will want to become total vegetarians — and that's probably not even advisable for serious athletes. But we can all benefit by cutting out those meats high in saturated fat and cholesterol. Start out by choosing leaner cuts, trimming off excess fat, and eating smaller portions — four ounces of meat will supply 30 grams of protein. Combining that with generous servings of several different vegetables can be just as appealing as a six-ounce cut with a baked potato. Also, try eating more fish and chicken. And for those of you who do want to follow a vegetarian lifestyle, you can substitute beans, eggs, nuts and vegetable-based protein supplements for meat as long as you meet your 30-gram target of protein for each meal. If you follow these recommendations, not only will you be getting less fat and cholesterol, but you'll be getting fewer calories as well. You'll look and feel better.

#3: Cut down on processed and convenience foods and eat more fresh fruits and vegetables. Today we eat less than half of the fresh fruits and vegetables that our grandparents did. We've largely replaced these foods with various processed and convenience foods. These processed and convenience foods are almost always lower in vitamins, minerals, and fiber and higher in calories, sugar, and fat. Rediscover the joys of fresh vegetables, lightly steamed, and served with just a trace of butter and a sprig of parsley. Choose raw vegetables, unsalted nuts and seeds, or fresh fruit for your snack foods. Drink water, real fruit juice (as opposed to "fruit-flavored" juice which is largely sugar water) or low fat milk for your beverages.

#4: Choose whole wheat whenever possible. Processing wheat removes 20 nutrients. "Enrichment" adds back only four. Whole grain products add significant amounts of vitamin E, vitamin B_6 (folic acid), magnesium, and zinc to your diet. In addition, whole wheat is an excellent natural source of fiber in your diet. Don't be fooled by misleading advertisements and labels. Unless it says 100% whole grain, it probably isn't.

#5: Cut down on the amount of sugar in your diet. Hidden sugar in the American diet is a major cause of obesity. Obesity, in turn, is the number one health problem in the United States today. Obesity is a major risk factor for diabetes, heart disease, high blood pressure, arthritis, and many other degenerative diseases. Never add sugar unless you absolutely have to. Avoid processed foods that are high in sugar (always read labels!). You'll find that desserts and snacks of fresh fruits in season will, in time, be just as appealing to you and your family as the sugary foods you now eat. Finally, simply add less sugar to the foods you cook. You'll find that most recipes will be sweet enough if you cut the amount of sugar in half. You can cut the amount you add in half again if you use honey or maple syrup because they are sweeter. Make these changes gradually and you'll find that your sweet tooth will diminish. You'll be satisfied with foods that are much less sweet and you'll rediscover many taste sensations that have been covered up by the excess sugar in your diet. Your waistline will thank you and your risk of developing serious disease will be lower.

#6: Cut down on the amount of salt in your diet. Excess salt causes hypertension (high blood pressure) in susceptible individuals. Unfortunately, there is no way to know if you are a susceptible individual until it is too late. Your best course of action is moderation in the use of salt. Simply avoid cured meats and salty foods. Natural sea salt contains far less sodium than processed table salt. Learn to use various combinations of herbs and spices rather than sugar and salt to liven up your cooking. Snack on fresh fruits or unsalted seeds or nuts in place of salty snack foods. Clinical trials show that you will lose your desire for salty foods in as few as two to three weeks. It's worth the effort.

#7: Use more monounsaturated and polyunsaturated oils to decrease the saturated fat and cholesterol in your diet. Oil and vinegar salad dressings are better for you. It is also easy to replace animal fats (e.g., lard) or hydrogenated vegetable fats (e.g., Crisco) with monounsaturated oils such as olive oil in your cooking. (You should remember, however, that if you sig-

nificantly increase your intake of polyunsaturated vegetable oils, you may need to increase your vitamin E intake.)

#8: Cut down on soft drinks and alcoholic beverages. These offer no nutrients, yet they have largely displaced milk and fruit juices from the American diet. Low fat milk remains our best source of calcium and 100 percent fruit juices are a good source of vitamin C and many other micronutrients.

#9: Avoid artificial and imitation foods whenever possible. They are often advertised as being low in cholesterol, low in fat or low in calories. While this sounds appealing, remember that these foods almost *never* contain all the nutrients of the foods they replace and many of them contain potential cancer-causing additives. There are over 3000 food additives in the American food supply today. The average adult eats 13 pounds of food additives each year. A number of food additives have been withdrawn from our food supply in recent years because new scientific research has shown that they are unsafe. Many other widely used additives are controversial, with major research studies suggesting that they may be toxic to the body. Still other additives have never been adequately tested. Many of the additives that you consume every day will be declared unsafe in the future. There is no need to be a human guinea pig. Simply take the time to read labels and avoid additive-laden foods. In almost every case, you can find a safer, additive-free food of similar nutritional value.

#10: Add a well-balanced supplement program for optimal health. We should all try to eat as well as we possibly can. Unfortunately, even with the best intentions, most of us will still fall far short of getting all the nutrients that our bodies need. The American lifestyle and food supply make it almost impossible for any but the most dedicated individuals to get adequate amounts of all the essential nutrients.

Nutritional Demands of an Athlete in Training

Why Protein? Our muscle fibers consist largely of protein, so protein is an important part of any athlete's diet, whether they are a professional athlete or a recreational athlete. Weight training and other kinds of vigorous exercise damage muscle fibers. We also break down some of our muscle protein during exercise as a source of energy. In addition, one of the main goals of any training program is to increase muscle mass because both strength and endurance will be re-

quired to perform well in a golf tournament or recreational sport.

Thus, one of the things that we need to do during the recovery period immediately after exercise is to replace the muscle protein that was lost during exercise and add new muscle to insure a net increase in muscle mass. The master hormone that drives this process is insulin, the same hormone that helps us keep our blood sugar levels under control. In addition, the essential amino acid leucine stimulates muscle protein synthesis, and the effects of insulin and leucine are synergistic. As you might suspect there is a window of time (two to four hours following exercise) when the muscle is maximally sensitized to the effects of both insulin and leucine. I will discuss how we optimize both insulin and leucine levels during that "recovery period" later in this chapter.

Why Carbohydrates? The most readily available source of energy during exercise, especially high intensity exercise, is the carbohydrate store in our muscle called glycogen. Glucose in our bloodstream is a secondary source of energy and can actually be used in preference to muscle glycogen stores when the intensity of exercise is low to moderate, a process called "glycogen sparing." Blood glucose initially comes from the carbohydrate content of recently eaten foods, next from glycogen stores in our liver and, as the liver glycogen stores begin to be depleted, from the breakdown of muscle protein.

You should think of carbohydrates as your source of both energy and endurance. The role of carbohydrates in providing energy is obvious since only muscle glycogen stores can efficiently fuel high intensity exercise. The role of carbohydrates in endurance is less obvious. If all you wanted to do was to finish a tournament or golf match you could rely on your fat stores (see below). However, if you need to turn it up a notch (increase the intensity of exercise) at the end of a long event, you will need your muscle glycogen stores to provide the energy that you need. In addition, your brain relies primarily on glucose as an energy source, so if you want mental clarity at the end of the match you will want to have maintained optimal blood glucose levels.

Thus, your strategy with respect to carbohydrates should be two-fold: to maximize your muscle and liver glycogen reserves between exercise sessions and to keep your blood sugar levels constant during exercise. The two- to four-hour window of high insulin sensitivity during the recovery period is the best time to maximize your muscle glycogen stores. Prior to and during the event carbohydrate-containing foods are important for maintaining sufficient blood glucose levels without depleting liver glyco-

gen or muscle protein stores. I will discuss specific strategies for achieving each of those goals later in this chapter.

Why Fat? Many trainers treat fats as something to be avoided at all cost. In fact, as long as the exercise is of low to moderate intensity, fats are a perfectly good energy source. And, training actually increases the ability of our muscles to use fat as an energy source. However, fats cannot support high intensity exercise and cannot be used as an energy source by the brain. That is why there is so much emphasis on carbohydrates as a source of muscle and liver glycogen reserves and on the importance of providing enough carbohydrates during exercise to keep blood sugar levels constant.

What Is the Ideal Diet Composition?

For weight maintenance and general health the big debate in recent years has been whether the diet should be low-fat and high-carbohydrate, or low-carbohydrate and high-fat. In terms of weight loss, there is not a dime's worth of difference between low-fat and low-carbohydrate diets if you follow them for a year or more. In terms of weight maintenance, the low-fat diets appear to fare a little better because of the caloric density of fats. However, most experts will tell you that it is not so much the relative amount of fats and carbohydrates; rather it is the type of fat and carbohydrate in the diet that is important.

Diets high in saturated fats and trans fats increase inflammation and tend to increase the risk of heart disease and certain cancers. That is why most experts recommend that we minimize saturated and trans fats and replace them with monounsaturated fats (from olive oil, peanuts, almonds and avocados), omega-6 polyunsaturated fats (from vegetable oils) and omega-3 polyunsaturated fats (from fish oil). Certain vegetable oils (flax seed and canola) are also rich in omega-3 fats, but the omega-3 fats contained in those vegetable oils are biologically much less active than the omega-3 fats in fish oils.

Diets high in simple sugars and refined grains tend to lead to elevations in blood sugar and triglycerides and may predispose one to diabetes, which is why most experts recommend that simple sugars be minimized and that refined grains be replaced with whole grains, fresh fruits and vegetables.

Protein appears to have been largely ignored in the debate as to whether diets should be low in fat or low in carbohydrates. The assumption has been that we don't need to worry about protein because most Americans get plenty of protein. However, recent research is challenging that assumption. It turns out that sarcopenia (loss of muscle mass) is a big problem, both during weight loss and as we age. Since muscle is metabolically very active, loss of muscle mass leads to a decrease in basal metabolic rate (the number of calories that we burn on a daily basis). That makes it more difficult to lose weight when dieting and increases the risk of obesity for people who are not trying to control calories. Some experts recommend that protein intake should be around 20 to 30 percent of calories rather than the 10 to 15 percent that most Americans currently get.

As with both fats and carbohydrates, some protein sources are healthier than others. Fatty meats are associated with a higher risk of both heart disease and cancer, and red meats appear to be associated with a higher risk of some cancers. This is why health experts tell us that we should emphasize vegetable protein sources, eggs and lean meats, especially fish and chicken.

What is the bottom line? While I would be the first to admit that there is no perfect diet composition, my personal recommendation is to aim for a diet that supplies around 40 to 45 percent of calories from healthy carbohydrates, 30 to 35 percent of calories from healthy fats and around 20 to 30 percent of calories from healthy proteins.

How Much Protein, Carbohydrates and Fat Should an Athlete Get From Their Diet?

Let's start by talking about protein recommendations. This is a debate that is as old as the field of sports nutrition and there is no definitive answer. I often find trainers recommending diets or supplements that are very high in protein and low in both carbohydrates and fat for increasing muscle mass. This doesn't make sense because athletes need carbohydrates to maintain optimal blood sugar levels and to properly use the protein in their diet. (Remember that, when our blood sugar levels fall, our body converts protein to glucose rather than using it to build muscle.)

On the other hand, the RDA recommendations for a person with a light to moderate activity level is 0.36 grams/pound of weight, which means that a 150-pound, relatively sedentary individual would be aiming for around 55 grams of protein each day. However, recent research shows that the RDA intake of protein may not be enough to maintain muscle mass, especially if you are over 50.

To understand the relationship between protein intake and maintenance of muscle mass, you need to know that muscle protein serves as an energy reserve for the body. We synthesize new muscle protein following each meal and we break it down as an energy source between meals and during exercise. The amount of muscle that we break down during fasting and exercise is pretty much fixed, so the maintenance of muscle mass is critically dependent on how much muscle protein we synthesize after each meal. An adult in their twenties will synthesize about half as much muscle protein following a meal with 15 to 20 grams of protein as they will following a meal with 30 grams of protein. Adults in their fifties will synthesize little or no muscle protein following a meal containing 15 grams of protein or less. They appear to require around 30 grams of protein at each meal to support muscle protein synthesis.

Thus, whether you are young or older, 30 grams of protein/meal appears to be optimal for preserving muscle mass. That would translate into around 0.6 grams of protein/pound of weight, and if you add in the extra protein required for an athlete with a vigorous activity level you are in the range of 0.7 to 0.8 grams of protein/pound of body weight. Thus, my recommendation is for around 0.6 to 0.8 grams of protein/pound of body mass unless you have kidney problems or are otherwise limited in the amount of protein you can consume.

As for carbohydrates and fats, the issue is not so much about the amount consumed as it is about the kinds of carbohydrates and fats consumed. The general guidelines of 40 to 45 percent healthy carbohydrates and 30 to 35 percent healthy fats apply to athletes just as much as they do to any other individual although there are some special issues with respect to the timing of carbohydrates and fats during exercise that I will describe later in this chapter.

The Importance of Water and Electrolytes Before and During the Event

Almost every athlete, whether professional or amateur, recognizes the importance of keeping adequately hydrated. As little as a two percent fluid loss will start to affect your performance. At four percent fluid loss, you will start to lose mental focus and may experience an increased heart rate. At six percent fluid loss, you may become disoriented, and at eight percent fluid loss you are likely to collapse. But water alone is not the best way to keep hydrated. That's because we lose electrolytes along with water when we sweat, and electrolytes are essential for muscle (including heart muscle) function and nerve conduction.

To understand why water alone is not the best option for keeping hydrated, you need to know that we have two fluid compartments in the body, our blood and our cells, and those two compartments equilibrate slowly. When we are sweating we lose water and electrolytes from both compartments. When we take a drink of water we rapidly dilute the concentration of electrolytes in the bloodstream and our thirst sensor signals that we are no longer dehydrated. But the cells are still dehydrated. It may take 10 or 15 minutes before the extra water in the bloodstream enters the cells and the electrolytes in the cells enter the bloodstream. Only then does our thirst sensor realize that we are still dehydrated and send a signal to our brain that we need to drink more fluid. So when we drink water alone we are constantly underestimating how much fluid we need to drink to maintain adequate hydration. But that's not the worst of it. Because electrolytes have been drawn from the cells into the bloodstream to maintain equilibrium between our two fluid compartments, the electrolyte levels in our cells can get too low for proper muscle and nerve function.

This is why most sports rehydration drinks contain electrolytes as well as water. Since it is important to start any event adequately hydrated and to maintain adequate hydration during the event, sports rehydration drinks should be consumed both before and during the event.

The Importance of Carbohydrates Before and During the Event

At the beginning of this chapter I talked about the importance of starting an event with adequate glycogen stores and maintaining optimal blood glucose levels during the event. That is why most sports drinks also provide carbohydrates and why carbohydrate-rich foods are generally recommended before and during the event. However, both the amount and type of carbohydrate in the sports drink are important considerations. The greater the carbohydrate content of the sports drink, the greater the endurance that it will support. The sports drink needs to contain some simple sugars because they get into the bloodstream very quickly. However, if the concentration of simple sugars in the sports drink is too high, it interferes with the ability of the stomach and intestine to absorb the water and electrolytes in the sports drink, leaving you feeling bloated and sluggish. A well-designed sports drink will contain a mixture of simple sugars for rapid uptake into the bloodstream and complex carbohydrates that will be taken into the bloodstream more slowly and will not interfere with uptake of water and electrolytes.

The Importance of Protein and Carbohydrates after the Event

As I mentioned earlier in this chapter, some trainers emphasize protein as if you only needed to replenish muscle protein after a workout or event. Others have emphasized carbohydrates (carbo loading) as if you only needed to replenish muscle glycogen.

In actuality a combination of protein and carbohydrate is needed to replenish the muscle protein and glycogen stores and to increase muscle mass. And when you consume both carbohydrate and protein together, you get a much greater insulin response than when you consume either of them alone.

Because both muscle protein synthesis and replenishing of muscle glycogen are driven by insulin and the effect of insulin is greatest right after the workout, post-workout meals or sports supplements should contain enough protein and carbohydrates to maximize the insulin response and should be consumed as soon as possible after exercise. Fifteen to 20 grams of protein and a carbohydrate ratio in the range of 2.5:1 to 3:1 appear to be optimal for maximizing the insulin response. And because leucine works synergistically with insulin to stimulate protein synthesis, protein sources that provide around 1.5 grams of leucine should be chosen.

However, the optimal amount of both leucine and protein appear to vary with age. For people in their twenties, 1.5 grams of leucine and 15 to 20 grams of protein seem to be adequate to support muscle protein synthesis. However, people in their fifties and above appear to need 2.5 to

3.0 grams of leucine and 30 grams of protein to stimulate muscle protein synthesis. Even people in their twenties will see a greater increase in muscle mass at 30 grams protein and 2.5 to 3.0 grams of leucine intakes than at 1.5 grams of leucine and 15 to 20 grams of protein. However, 30 grams of protein will probably be best utilized if it is not consumed all at once. Thus, I recommend that 15 to 20 grams of protein supplying around 1.5 grams of leucine and enough carbohydrates to maximize the insulin response be consumed immediately after the workout or event, and an additional protein-rich meal or sports supplement be consumed one to two hours later to supply the rest of the protein and leucine needed to rebuild and increase muscle mass.

Omega-3s for Inflammation

Inflammation is an inevitable part of sports. Whether you are a professional athlete who is continually pushing yourself to the limit or the weekend warrior who only exercises in spurts, you will experience pain and inflammation from time to time. While there are many natural approaches that can give you quick and temporary pain relief, a diet rich in omega-3 fats is the best way to "dial down" the inflammatory response in your body so that you will be less likely to develop pain and inflammation. The polyun-

saturated fats in our diet are incorporated into our cell membranes unchanged (This is the one case where it is literally true that we are what we eat). Whenever we damage our muscles or ligaments during exercise, the polyunsaturated fats in our cell membranes are converted to hormone-like substances called prostaglandins. The polyunsaturated fats in the typical American diet are converted to pro-inflammatory prostaglandins, while the omega-3 polyunsaturated fats are converted to anti-inflammatory prostaglandins. It's a simple concept. We can't always avoid the sprains and strains of exercise, but we can control how our cells respond to those sprains and strains just by increasing the amount of omega-3 fats in our diet.

But there are many kinds of omega-3 fats, and not just any omega-3 fat source will do. Omega-3 fats from vegetable source are converted to the anti-inflammatory prostaglandins with only about 10 percent of the efficiency of omega-3 fats from fish. So fish would seem to be the logical choice, but unfortunately our oceans are polluted. For example, the Environment Protection Agency has recommended that maximum consumption of most wild salmon range between once a week to once a month because of contamination with PCBs and heavy metals.

Farm-raised fish are even worse. The Environmental Protection Agency recommends that some farm-raised salmon be consumed no more than once a year. So that seems to leave fish oil supplements as the preferred choice for omega-3 fats. But you need to know that the food supplement industry is unregulated. For example, in March 2010 the Mateel Environmental Group sued the manufacturer and distributors of 90 percent of the fish oil supplements in California because their fish oil products were contaminated with PCBs. I love salmon and choose wild salmon whenever I can get it, but my recommendation for daily use is to choose an ultrapure fish oil supplement from a manufacturer that you can trust.

Sports Nutrition Supplements: The Good, the Bad & the Ugly

Many athletes are looking for an edge, and there are a lot of unscrupulous sports nutrition manufacturers who are just trying to rip off the gullible. So before I summarize my recommendations, I will just make a few comments about the supplements that are illegal, dangerous, completely bogus or simply not supported by strong science.

The Illegal: Hopefully, everyone reading this chapter knows that steroids and amphetamines are both dangerous and illegal.

Ephedrine, ephedra or ma huang can increase alertness but don't actually enhance performance. Even worse, they can cause an increase in blood pressure and heart rate. These supplements have actually killed people so they are currently banned by the FDA.

The Dangerous: Growth hormone, DHEA and other pro-hormones are effective at increasing muscle mass. While many athletes naively assume that they are safe, DHEA and related pro-hormones are precursors to the steroid hormones, so they can have some of the same dangerous side effects that steroids have. Even worse, all of these hormones stimulate the growth of cancer cells, so there is a real concern that long-term use may increase cancer risk.

And finally there are the amino acid supplements that certain manufacturers claim will increase levels of growth hormone, DHEA or other hormones. The evidence that these amino acid supplements actually work is very sparse, and, if they did work, I would have the same concerns as with the hormones themselves.

The Bogus: Ribose has a very specific beneficial effect for heart disease patients, but there is no evidence that it provides any exercise benefit in healthy individuals.

Carnitine shows little or no beneficial effects on exercise in clinical studies, and some studies have cast doubt on whether it is even taken up by muscle cells.

HMB is a metabolite of leucine. It has been claimed to increase levels of growth hormone, but most clinical studies have not supported that claim. Even worse, excessive use of HMB has been reported to lead to confusion and memory loss.

Arginine has been claimed to increase levels of nitric oxide. If that were true, it might be of some benefit because nitric oxide opens up blood vessels, thus potentially increasing the flow of oxygen and nutrients to the muscle. However, clinical studies have not supported the claim that supplemental arginine can increase nitric oxide levels.

A Special Case: Caffeine can increase heart rate and cause palpitations, so it is not completely benign. However, millions of Americans already use caffeine in some form (coffee, tea, soft drinks) every day, and clinical studies show that it increases alertness and has a modest effect on endurance. So if you tolerate caffeine well, there is no reason not to use it. However, I am not a big fan of the many energy drinks and energy products in the marketplace today because they generally contain artificial flavors, colors, sweeteners and preservatives. I exercise to improve my health, so I don't want to be putting those kinds of things in my body. If you want to add caffeine to your exercise routine, I recommend getting it from a food (coffee or tea) or caffeine supplement without artificial ingredients.

My Recommendations: It all starts with a healthy diet. We need to assure that we are getting the nutrients that we need on a daily basis from foods that will support our health and our athletic endeavors. The ten steps to a healthy diet that I listed at the beginning of this chapter are a good guideline, but they are only a guideline. In today's world we are often presented with unhealthy food choices, especially if we do a lot of traveling. So that is why I recommend using a good food supplement on a daily basis as well.

If you want to maintain or increase muscle mass, you will probably need to increase your protein intake above the currently recommended levels. I recommend aiming for 0.6 to 0.8 grams of protein per pound of weight per day. The bulk of this protein should be healthy protein: lean white meats and vegetable protein, and it should be fairly evenly distributed between all three meals.

To maximize your endurance, you should use a rehydration product before and during your event. Chose a product that contains both electrolytes and carbohydrate – a mixture of simple sugar and complex carbohydrate is best. Easily digestible, carbohydrate-rich foods (bananas, for example) can also be consumed during the event. And, once again, try to avoid rehydration products that contain artificial ingredients. My motto is, "If it comes in blue, don't use it."

To maximize the recovery process, you should make sure that you consume both carbohydrates and protein in an easily digestible form immediately after your workout or event. Aim for 15 to 20 grams of protein and a ratio range of carbohydrate to protein of 2.5:1 to 3:1 to maximize the insulin response. Follow that up with a meal or sports nutrition supplement within the next one to two hours to bring your total post-workout protein intake to around 30 grams. That will generally also bring your total leucine intake to around 2 to 3 grams. Don't go crazy trying to optimize the amounts and ratios. There are sports nutrition supplements that will help you reach these targets easily. You shouldn't need to be a math whiz to be a successful athlete.

To minimize inflammation, make sure that your diet contains plenty of omega-3 fats. Unless your inflammation is severe, 500 to 1000 mg of omega-3 fats should be plenty. Fish oil is superior to vegetable sources of the omega-3 fats, and until problems with contamination of our fish supply can be overcome, I recommend that you rely on an ultra-pure fish oil supplement from a manufacturer that you can trust.

Part 4

Understanding the Exercises

FOLLOWING IS A list and categories of the exercises used for my workout programs. These are my staple exercises and there are many more that I could include. If you have a favorite exercise that is missing from my list, feel free to add or substitute it to the corresponding workout as long as they fit into the philosophy laid out in this book and as long as you perform that exercise with the use of the same principles as explained. I don't have any "miracle" exercises; the difference lies in the way the exercise is performed as explained previously.

Look carefully at the description and details for each exercise. It is important that you understand and follow them. Each exercise is accompanied by a column containing an explanation as well as possible variations and progressions, all designed to enhance speed, balance, and stability.

Remember even though these exercises are categorized into their respective body parts, you will always want to distribute the loads through the whole body. Plus there is always a certain amount of a crossover, i.e the arms are also involved in pushups and pullups.

Strength: This refers to the amount of weight or resistance that can be used in different phases of the workout on a scale of light to medium to heavy to maximum compared to the one repetition maximum.

I do not recommend trying to determine your one rep max on your own without the help of a trainer; neither do I recommend exceeding 90 percent of your maximum without a trainer supervising you. (The difference in doing an exercise at 90 percent of maximum versus 100 percent of maximum does not warrant enough gains to risk injury.)

Light = 20-30% of max
Medium = 30-60% of max
Heavy = 60-80% of max
Max = 80-100% of max

Speed: is on a scale ranging from **static** to **slow** to **medium** to **high,** and **rhythmic** and can be different depending on the phase you are in. The weight has to be adjusted accordingly (lighter) for fast and rhythmic. It is important that not to sacrifice perfect form for speed.

Static = no movement.

Slow = two-count on the concentric and four-count on the eccentric.

Medium = one count on the concentric and two-count on the eccentric.

High = as fast as possible on the concentric and two-count on the eccentric.

Rhythmic = concentric and eccentric are at about equal speed from medium to high, with a rhythm close to the golf swing and the acceleration and deceleration being gradual (think of a pendulum here).

Balance: progressions will be described as ranging from doing the exercise with **feet close together** to doing them on **one foot** to doing them on the **balance board** (normal would be your stance as described in "The Base")

Stability: is partially dependent on balance but depends mostly on strength and the ability to connect the body with the progressions being described as taking away stability, like **one leg** or **one arm** or both or **adding a physio ball** or **balance board.**

Abbreviations used:

KAI FUSSER

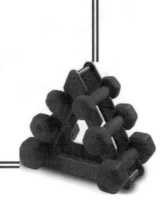

Abbreviations used:

DB = Dumb Bell

BB = Bar Bell

RB = Rubber Band

MD = Medicine Ball

PB = Physio Ball

IB = Indoboard™

FR = Foam Roller

WEIGHT TRAINING FOR GOLF

The arms are the first connection with the club. They also act as extra leverage. It is important to have strong arms. At the same time, you want to learn to relax them in order to transfer power through them to the club and not to inhibit the flow.

1.　Twisting biceps curl

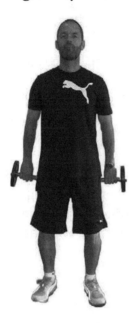 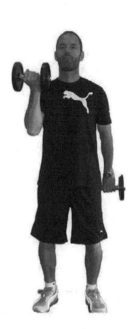

This curl recruits the biceps in its full capacity for bending and rotating the forearm.

Start with a loose grip and your palms facing back behind your hips. Twist and curl to top with a full range of motion in both positions. Keep the palms facing up while lowering the DBs.

Resistance	Speed	Balance	Stability
Light	**Slow**		**One foot**
Max	**Medium**		**1B**

2. One arm twisting biceps curl to overhead alternating

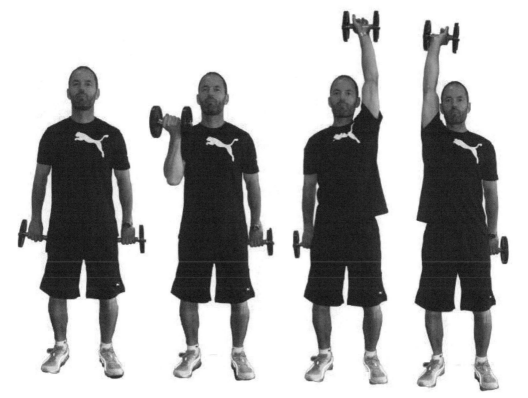

This one arm overhead version will require more stabilization from your core in order to stay aligned. Can be done alternating with a seamless transition and rhythm.

Start with a loose grip and palm facing back. Twist and curl with full extension to top position while keeping the body aligned. Keep the palm facing up while lowering the DB.

Resistance	Speed	Balance	Stability
Light	**Slow**		**One foot**
Heavy	**Medium**		**IB**
	Rhythm		

KAI FUSSER

3. Cable concentration curl

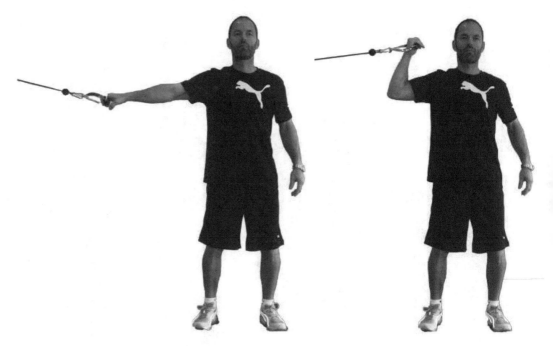

This is a great exercise to learn how to let forces flow. When done right, you will feel that your core will do most of the work and also has to stabilize your body to prevent it from bending.

With the cable at shoulder height, start with the arm relaxed and fully extended. Curl while keeping the elbow in line with the cable and the wrist straight. Feel the abs helping with the pull, letting the forces flow through your arm.

Resistance	Speed	Balance	Stability
Light ↓ Max	Slow		Feet together
Max	Medium		1 Foot (inside)

4. One arm cable curl

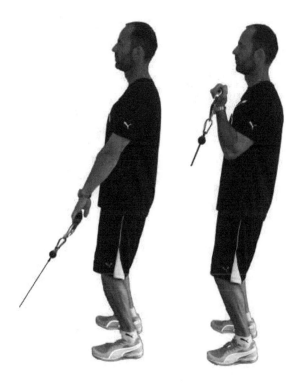

Stand close to the cable column. With a loose grip and the palm facing down, let the cable stretch your arm. Curl the handle up while also rotating the fore-arm. Resist bending the upper body by engaging the abs.

Resistance	Speed	Balance	Stability
Light	Slow		One leg
Heavy	Medium		IB

5. Hammer curl to overhead extension

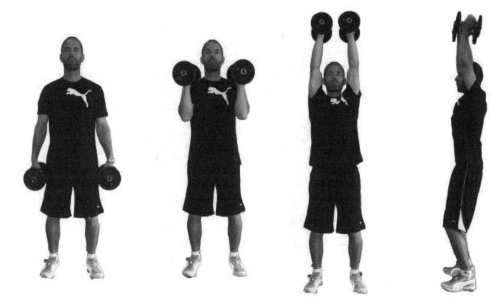

One of my favorites for upper body strength, it can be done in almost every variation, from light to max, with static or pumping legs (up and down), slow, fast and with rhythm, on one leg or using a IB, or in combination. You can even add a squat to it and turn it into a full body exercise.

With the DBs parallel to each other and a loose grip, curl the DBs to the shoulder position and then to the fully extended position. Try to reach the ceiling and feel the connection from the hands down to your feet.

Resistance	Speed	Balance	Stability
Light	Slow		One foot
Max	High		IB
	Rhythm		

6. Triceps kickback

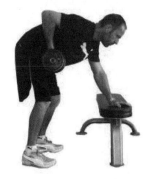 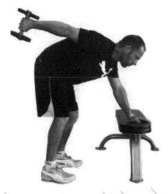

Through the rotation of the forearm this is one of the most complete triceps exercises

With upper body parallel to the ground, bent knees, elbow up and palm facing forward, kick the DB back to extended position while turning the hand 90 degrees without dropping the elbow.

Resistance	Speed	Balance	Stability
Light ↓ Heavy	Slow		
	Medium		

7. Cable triceps extension abducted

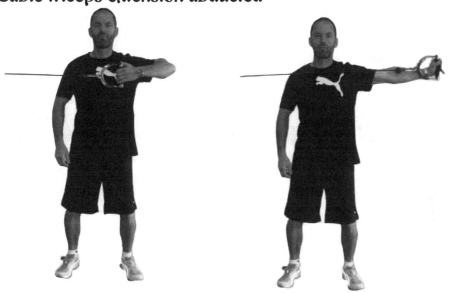

This exercise builds also a great connection between the triceps and the shoulder, which also improves the stabilization of the arm.

Start with elbow abducted in line with the cable. Without moving the elbow, fully extend the arm.

Resistance	Speed	Balance	Stability
Light	Slow		Feet together
Medium	Medium		One foot

8. Cable triceps pushdown

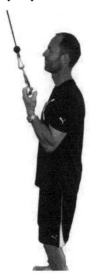 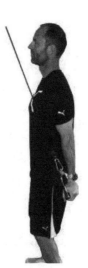

Stay close to the cable column. Start with a loose grip and the palm facing up. The elbow can be slightly in front of your body in the starting position. Extend the forearm down with a slight rotation of your hand. Make sure not to dip the shoulder in order to help the push down.

Resistance	Speed	Balance	Stability
Light	**Slow**		**One foot**
Medium	**Medium**		

9. Rope triceps pushdown

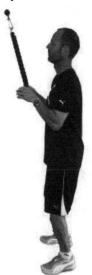 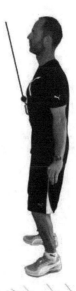

Great triceps exercise to use heavy weights. Stay close to the cable column. Start with your elbows slightly in front of your body and push down to the fully extended position. Make sure to keep your spine straight and don't use your shoulders to help push down.

Resistance	Speed	Balance	Stability
Light	Slow		Feet together
Max	Medium		One foot

10. Chin-ups

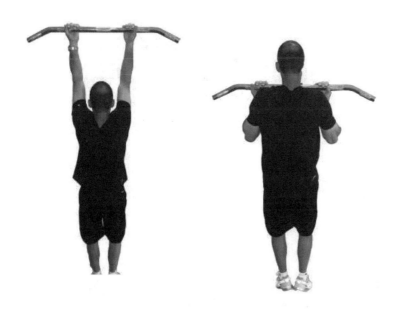

This is a great exercise for strength as well as for building a good connection between your hands and your torso. Keep a loose grip and pull your chin toward the bar, and lower your body slowly. You can use your legs for help as necessary on the way up as well as down.

Resistance	Speed	Balance	Stability
Body weight	Slow		
Heavy	Medium		

KAI FUSSER

11. Close grip pushups

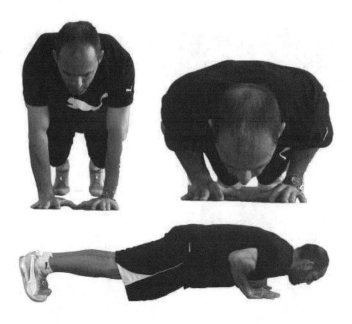

This exercise builds a strong connection between you triceps through the shoulders and chest to the core. With a close grip, keep your elbows close to your side, keeping your abs and gluteus engaged to maintain a straight body. Lower slowly as far as your strength allows, and then push up with the help of your abs by pulling your midsection toward the ceiling.

Resistance	Speed	Balance	Stability
Body weight	**Slow**		**One leg**
	Medium		

SHOULDERS

The shoulders are the main connecters between the arms and the chest and back muscles; they are also responsible for stabilizing the arms. Get strong shoulders to prevent very common shoulder injuries from the repetitive stress of the swing.

1. DB rotation exterior up

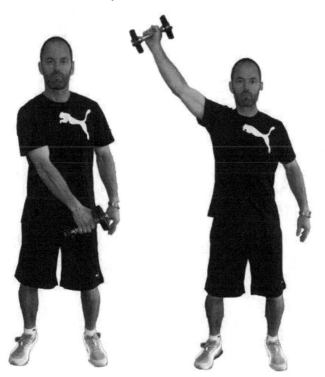

Great for shoulder stability, strength and gain of range of motion, it will also teach you to stay aligned despite the load from the side. With extended (not locked) arm, bring the DB to the top position to full range of motion without turning the upper body.

Resistance	Speed	Balance	Stability
Light	Slow		One foot
Medium	Medium		IB

KAI FUSSER

2. DB rotation interior up

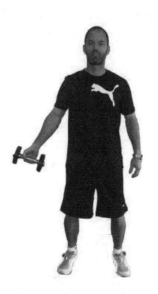 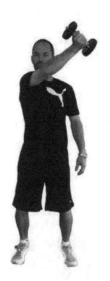

Here you can feel great help from your abs when engaged. Start with arm extended (not locked) and bring DB to top position without turning or leaning the head or shoulders. Try to bring your biceps to your chin.

Resistance	Speed	Balance	Stability
Light	**Slow**		**One foot**
Medium	**Medium**		**IB**

3. Cable rotation exterior down

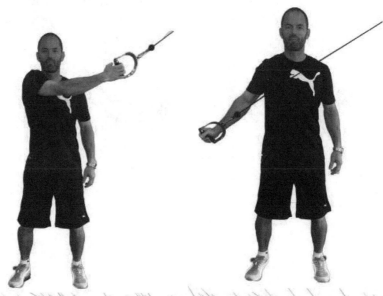

I really like this shoulder exercise as it helps with gaining range of motion while getting stronger and also teaches you to recruit the abs for help. With the cable at its highest position, start with a loose grip and stretched shoulder. Keep arm straight (not locked) and come down in front of your body to extended position. Return slowly in front of your body and feel how the engaged abs control the speed.

Resistance	Speed	Balance	Stability
Light	Slow		Feet together
Medium	Medium		One foot (inside)
	Rhythm		

4. Cable rotation interior down

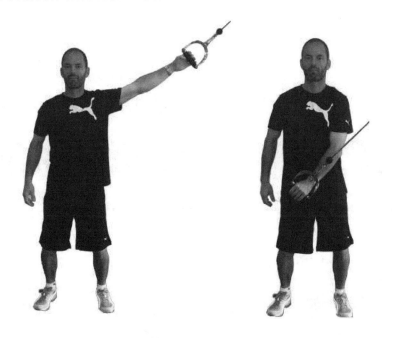

Start with a loose grip and stretched shoulder. Keep arm straight (not locked) and come down in front of your body to the extended position without rotating the shoulder.

Resistance	Speed	Balance	Stability
Light	Slow		Feet together
Medium	Medium		One foot

5. DB rotation neutral

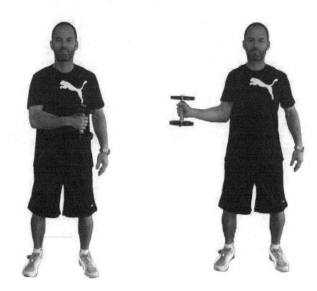

This exercise is important for the strengthening of the rotator cuff and increasing range of motion. You should be able to rotate the forearm about 90 degrees out from your body. Keep elbow at 90 degrees and close to the body. Rotate to full range of motion while keeping the elbow tucked in.

Resistance	Speed	Balance	Stability
Light	**Slow**		

6. DB rotation abducted

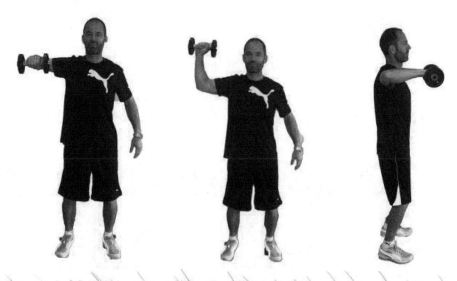

Complements the neutral rotation. With elbow abducted and at 90 degrees, rotate arm from the horizontal to the vertical position while keeping the elbow still.

Resistance	Speed	Balance	Stability
Light	**Slow**		

7. DB overhead extension

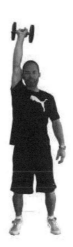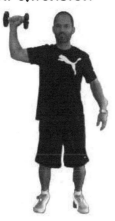

This extension works great to build strength and open up the shoulder. It is also great for connecting your hands to your feet while staying aligned. Start with elbow at 90 degrees and bring DB to top position while fully extending the arm, without leaning of the head or shoulders.

Resistance	Speed	Balance	Stability
Light	**Low**		**One leg**
Heavy	**Medium**		**IB**

8. DB rotation exterior up alternating

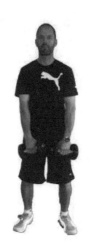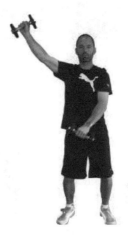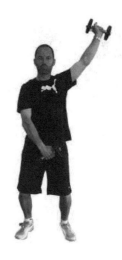

This alternating version will require you to use your abs extensively, especially when creating some rhythm. With loose grip and arms slightly crossed, alternately lift the arms to the extended position. When adding rhythm, use the legs in a up and down pumping motion to get free of the weight (the DB will seem lighter).

Resistance	Speed	Balance	Stability
Light	Slow		One leg
Medium	Rhythm		IB

9. DB rotation interior up alternating

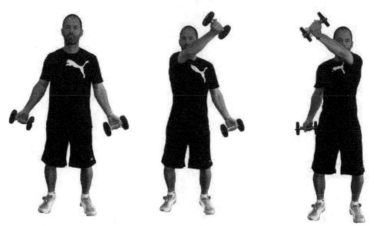

Same as with the exterior version, making sure your biceps comes toward the chin.

Resistance	Speed	Balance	Stability
Light	Slow		One leg
Medium	Rhythm		IB

10. DB front to side raises alternating

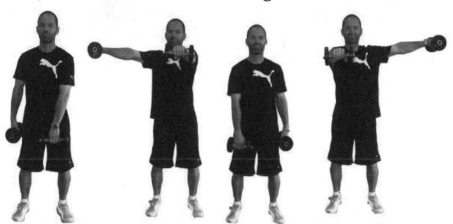

I love exercises where you can build strength and coordination at the same time and this is one of them. Keep a loose grip and start with one arm facing forward and the other arm facing to the side. Lift both DBs at the same time with the help of your abs and the up and down pumping motion of your legs. Try to use your shoulders as little as possible. Repeat while alternating the positions of the arms. If the coordination and timing is right, feel how the weight of the DB seems to almost disappear, getting free of the weight.

Resistance	Speed	Balance	Stability
Light	Slow		One leg
Medium	Rhythm		IB

11. Lying rear deltoid

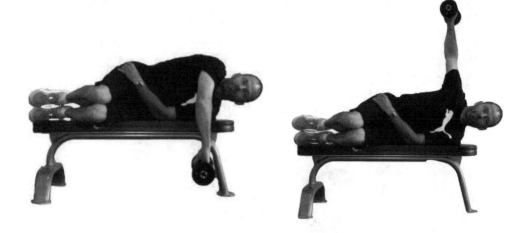

Lying on your side, let the arm be stretched by the DB with the palm facing toward your feet. With help from your abs, lift to the top position right above your shoulder. Be careful to not go too far back as it can make you fall off the bench.

Resistance	Speed	Balance	Stability
Light	**Slow**		
Medium			

12. Cable rotation neutral

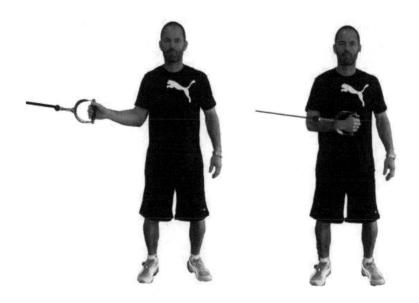

Just like the DB version, this exercise is great for rotator cuff strength and maintenance. The constant pull from the cable will help with increasing range of motion. Stand sideways to the cable column and keep the elbow close to your side. Feel a stretch from the pull of the cable (no pain!) and rotate in; return slowly.

Resistance	Speed	Balance	Stability
Light	Slow		

13. Cable rotation abducted

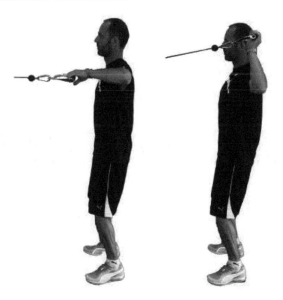

Stand facing the cable column with the cable at shoulder height. Rotate the forearm up to the 90-degree position while keeping the elbow still; return slowly.

Resistance	Speed	Balance	Stability
Light	Slow		

14. Cable front deltoid

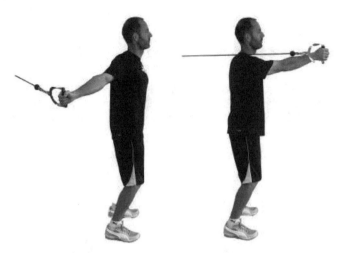

With the cable at shoulder height and arm straight (not locked), face away from the cable column. Without turning the shoulders, let the arm reach back without getting too much of a stretch (no pain!). With the help of the abs, rotate the arm to the front position and return slowly.

Resistance	Speed	Balance	Stability
Light	Slow		

15. Cable rear deltoid

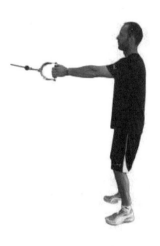 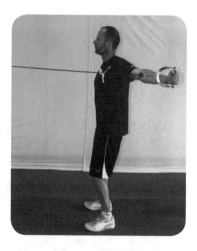

Facing the cable column. With the arm fully extended (not locked), rotate the arm back as far as possible without much of a shoulder rotation; return slowly.

Resistance	Speed	Balance	Stability
Light	Slow		

CHEST

Just like the back muscles, the chest muscles connect the shoulders to the core. They also are important to stabilize the connection between the shoulders and arms

1. Flat bench DB chest press together

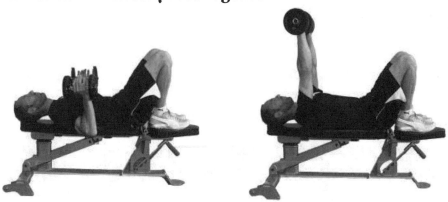

This is still one of the good old chest exercises. Start with elbows level to the bench and your feet up. With help by drawing your abs toward the bench, push the DB up to a fully extended position (not locked) right above the shoulders with a 90-degree rotation and return slowly.

Resistance	Speed	Balance	Stability
Light	Slow		PB
Max	Medium		

KAI FUSSER

2. Incline bench DB chest press togeth

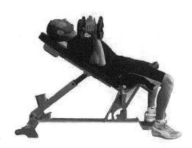 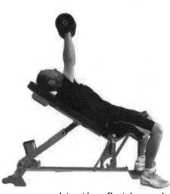

This will require more help from your shoulders, compared to the flat bench version. With the bench at 30 degrees, start with elbows level to the bench. Draw abs to bench and push DB up with a 90-degree rotation to a fully extended position (not locked) right above the shoulders and return slowly.

Resistance	Speed	Balance	Stability
Light	Slow		
Max	Medium		

3. Incline bench DB chest press alternating

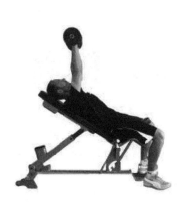 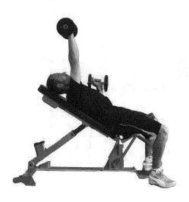

Same as the together version, but alternating the pressing arm. Keep a loose grip and create a good rhythm.

Resistance	Speed	Balance	Stability
Light	Slow		
Medium	Medium		
Heavy	Rhythm		

4. Incline BB press

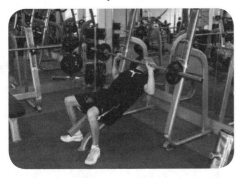 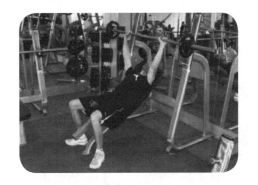

BB bench presses are great for building strength and power as well as building a connection between your arms and torso. As the arms are connected through the bar, you can use much more weight than when using DB's. Also, by connecting your arms the shoulders now turned into a hinge joint vs. a ball joint which requires less stabilization... Grab the bar just past shoulder width, and then lower slowly until the bar is about 3 to 4 inches from your chest. Draw abs to the bench and push up to a fully extended position (not locked) above the shoulders. Use a spotter for this exercise when using heavy weights..

Resistance	Speed	Balance	Stability
Light	Slow		
↓ Heavy	Medium		

KAI FUSSER

5. Flat bench BB chest press

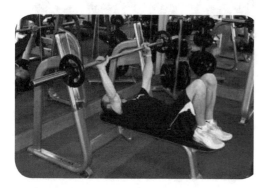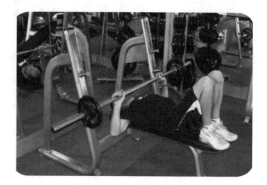

Grab the bar just past shoulder width, lower slowly until the bar is about 3 to 4 inches from your chest. Draw abs toward the bench and push up to a fully extended position (not locked) above the shoulders. Use a spotter for this exercise when using heavy weights.

Resistance	Speed	Balance	Stability
Light	**Slow**		
Max	**Medium**		
	High		

WEIGHT TRAINING FOR GOLF

6. Bent arm pull over

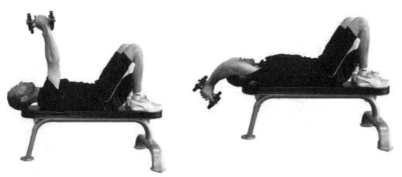

This one is great as a stretching exercise and also to feel and build the connection between your hands and abs. Lie with your head near the end of the bench. With the arms slightly bent, lower the weight slowly to a comfortable stretch position, draw abs into the bench and raise the arms back up. You should feel that the abs are pulling the weight up rather than the arms.

Resistance	Speed	Balance	Stability
Light	**Slow**		

7. Lying rope pull over

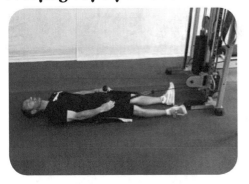 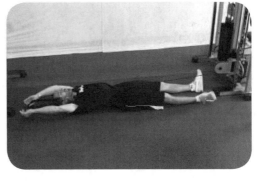

Lie flat on the floor and extend your arms to the cable. Pull the rope overhead with the help of your abs. Alternate between the left and right sides of your head and return slowly.

Resistance	Speed	Balance	Stability
Light	**Slow**		
Heavy	**Medium**		

8. Cable cross over

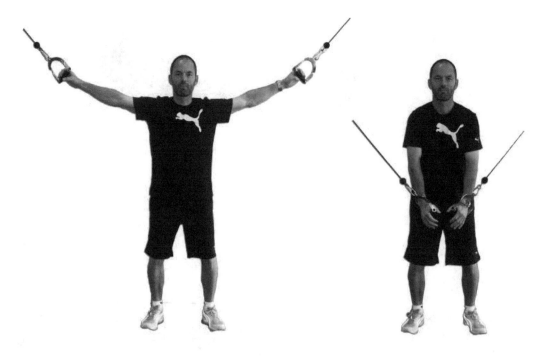

Good stretch and connection exercises. With the cable set high, let the weight take you into a comfortable stretch. Bring arms together just in front of your body; return slowly.

Resistance	Speed	Balance	Stability
Light	**Slow**		
Heavy	**Medium**		

9. Pushups

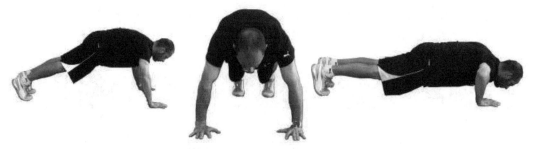

This is still one of the best. I see a pushup more as a core and connection exercise than a pure chest exercise. Make sure you create and feel the connection between your hands and feet. Think of a pushup as being a plank that moves up and down. With abs and gluteus engaged, lower the whole body slowly. Initiate the upward movement by drawing the abs up toward the ceiling as if you are pulling yourself up via your belly button. As you can see, there are many progressions to a pushup. Make sure you always feel in control of your core. Stop if you lose your back (turning into a reverse C).

Resistance	Speed	Balance	Stability
Light	Slow		One leg
Medium	Medium		Hands on IB
Heavy	Fast		Feet on PB
Max			IB + PB

10. Pushups wide

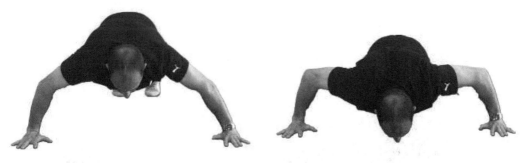

This will work the shoulders more.

Resistance	Speed	Balance	Stability
Light	Slow		One leg
Heavy	Fast		Legs on PB

11. Pushups with weight

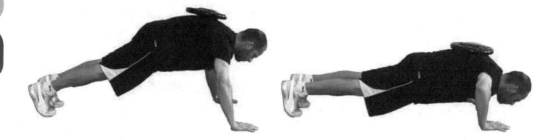

This brings a new meaning to pushups. (Annika did three with 80 pounds!)
It is critical to use the abs correctly to support the extra weight on your back.

Resistance	Speed	Balance	Stability
Light ↓	Slow		One leg
Max	Medium		Legs on PB
			Hands on IB

12. Pushups on ball shins

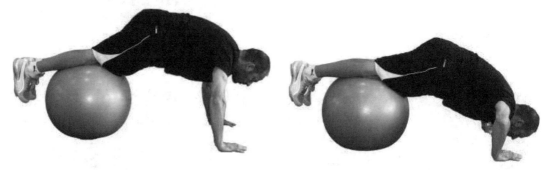

The easiest way to start on the ball.

Resistance	Speed	Balance	Stability
Light	Slow		Hands on IB
Medium	Medium		

13. Pushups on ball, two feet

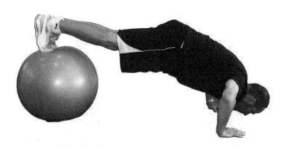

Start with the feet flat at first and then later try lifting up onto the toes. Control your balance using your abs.

Resistance	Speed	Balance	Stability
Light	**Slow**		**Hands on IB**
Medium	**Medium**		
Heavy	**Fast**		

14. Pushups on ball, one foot

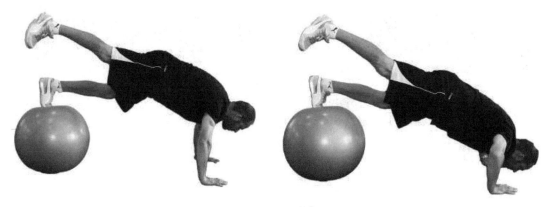

When mastered, try alternating the feet while moving.

Resistance	Speed	Balance	Stability
Light	**Slow**		**Hands on IB**
Medium	**Medium**		
Heavy	**Fast**		

KAI FUSSER

BACK

The back muscles are a big power producer in the swing and also act as the main connecters between the shoulders and the hips.

1. Bent over DB rowing

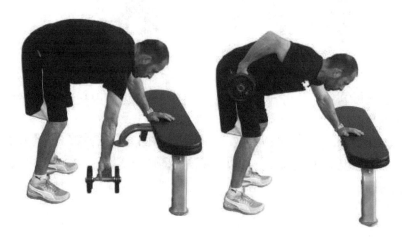

With upper body parallel to the floor, use a loose grip with palm facing out, and let the DB stretch your upper back and down your lats. Pull the elbow back and upward using the lats. Keep a loose grip and turn palm facing forward. Make sure you keep the abs engaged to protect your back.

Resistance	Speed	Balance	Stability
Light	Slow		
Heavy	Medium		

2. Standing row

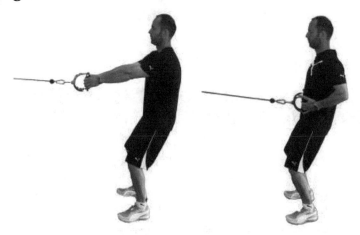

Why do this sitting when you can stand up? This really builds a good connection between the hands and the feet. Start with the arms and upper body stretched toward the cable. Keep a loose grip. While pulling the handle in toward the belly, draw the scapular back and push the chest out. Return slowly.

Resistance	Speed	Balance	Stability
Light	Slow		One leg
↓			
Max	Medium		

3. Jockey row

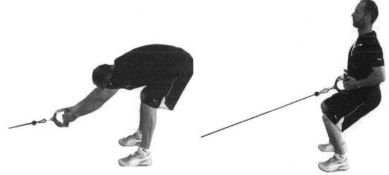

With the jockey row you will learn how to balance out the high forces of the pull from the cable so not to get pulled forward or not to fall back. If the forces from the top and bottom meet at the center of your body (just below the belly button) you will be able to handle quite some weight in balance.

With the cable low and using a loose grip, let the weight put you into a comfortable stretch with the thighs at about 45 degrees to the floor. Engage abs and bring the upper body upright while pulling the handle in toward the belly and sit into a squat position. Draw the scapular back and push the chest out; return slowly.

Resistance	Speed	Balance	Stability
Light	Slow		One leg
↓			
Max	Medium		

KAI FUSSER

WEIGHT TRAINING FOR GOLF

4. Pullups

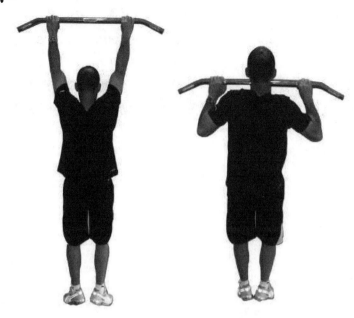

This is still my favorite and may be the best exercise to build a connection between your hands and the core. It will build the lats, which are most important connectors for transferring power from the core to the club's shaft. This is especially important for power shots like getting out of the deep rough. (Annika ended up doing 15 "clean" pullups. She also used a weight belt!) Pullups are much harder for women than men, as men's bodies contain more muscle fibers in the upper body. There are different progressions to do pullups: you can start at your strength level and work your way up. It may not be much fun but I can promise you they will pay off. Start with arms extended and keep a loose grip. Maintain a slight tension in the shoulders and pull yourself up by engaging the back; lower slowly. Even here you want to keep a loose grip and relax your body.

Resistance	Speed	Balance	Stability
Light ↓	Slow		
Max	Medium		
	Fast		

5. Pullups on straps angled

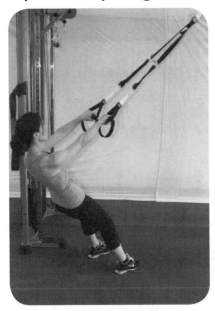 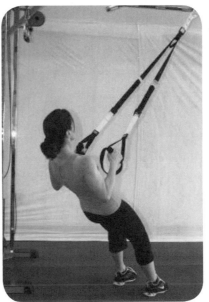

Remember that the more upright you are, the less weight you have to pull. Keep moving further under the rope as you get stronger.

6. Pullups with leg help

As an alternative, a bench can be placed under the feet to help by using the legs to raise and lower the body. Start with the feet right underneath you and use the legs as much as needed. Now you can make it as hard as you want by using the legs less and pulling more with upper body. At some point you may be able to jump up and take your feet off the ground for part of the way down and "catch" yourself with your legs just before you get to the low position. (don't fall into the shoulders!)

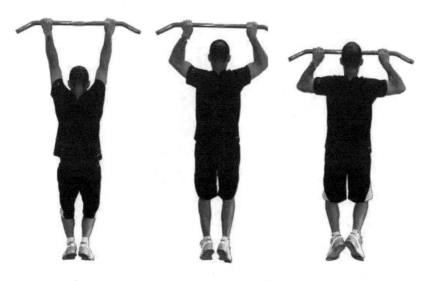

7. Pullups with helper

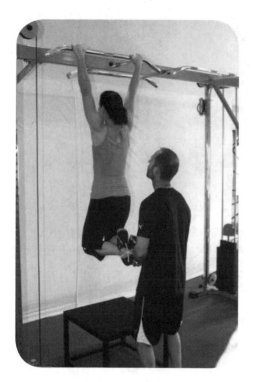 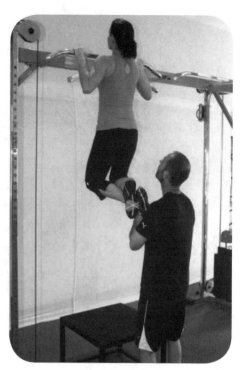

The helper can help you on the way up as much as needed and less on the way down as you are stronger during the eccentric movement. This is a much better way compared to using a assisted pullup machine as the machine also helps you on the way down so you are missing out on the important eccentric load.

8. Pullups on straps

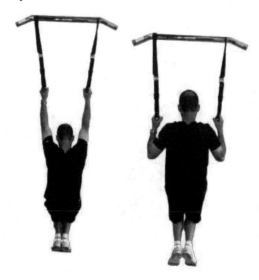

These are a little harder than on the bar, as the shoulders are moving more freely and therefore have to stabilize more.

Resistance	Speed	Balance	Stability
Light	Slow		
Medium	Medium		
Heavy	Fast		

9. Pullups on straps parallel grip

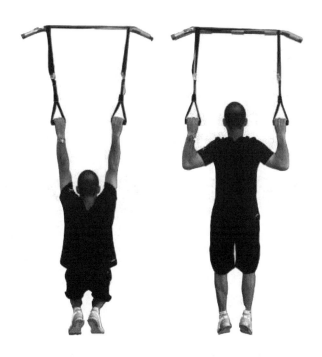

Another variation, this is the easiest on the shoulders by keeping the hands parallel to each other.

Resistance	Speed	Balance	Stability
Light	Slow		
Medium	Medium		
Heavy	Fast		

10. Cable lat pull down

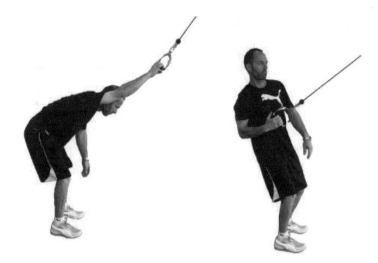

With a loose grip, let the cable stretch the arms and lats. Start by bringing the upper body up and rotating the shoulders. Pull the handle with the lats while keeping the forearm aligned with the cable. If you see the wrist curling, that means you are pulling too much with your arm.

Resistance	Speed	Balance	Stability
Light	**Slow**		**One leg**
Medium	**Medium**		
Heavy	**Rhythm**		

11. Rope lat pull down alternating

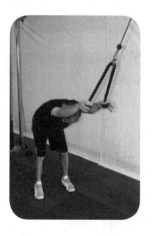 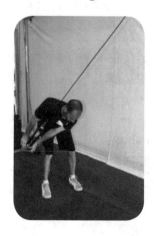 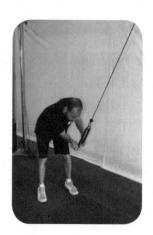

Builds the connection between your hands through the lats to the core. Start with a loose grip and arms extended. Feel a comfortable stretch. Engage the abs and pull the straight (not locked) arms alternating to each side.

Resistance	Speed	Balance	Stability
Light	Slow		One leg
Medium	Medium		
Heavy	Rhythm		

12. Kneeling two-arm lat pull down

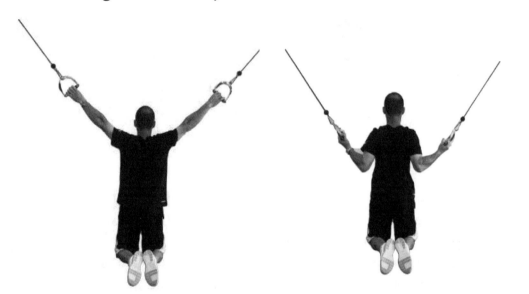

Another good one for connecting the hands to the torso through the lats. With the cable in the high position, feel a comfortable stretch. With a loose grip, draw the arms down by using your lats, bringing the elbows to your side. Squeeze the shoulder blades together and return slowly.

Resistance	Speed	Balance	Stability
Light ↓ Heavy	Slow		
	Medium		

LEGS

Your legs may be strong already but they can never be strong enough. These exercises will strengthen all the stabilizing muscles in your legs which will protect your joints and create stability. The legs are invaluable for power production and stabilization. With these exercises you will not only build strength but also learn how to incorporate your leg muscles within every move.

1. Front lunge

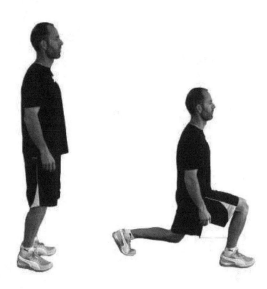

Lunges are still one of the best exercises for leg strength, building stability in the ankles, knees and hips and increasing balance. Lunges are also a great way to practice the reengagement of the abs just before the change of direction and push back up. This is the same type of directional change as in the transition between the back swing and the down swing. You can create approximately the same timing as in the swing. Step forward while keeping the knee over the foot. The back leg stays loose. Initiate the push up with the front leg. Reengage the abs just before the push up to the starting position. With all lunges, make sure that your knee does not move past your toes. Try to sit into your gluteus as much as possible.

Resistance	Speed	Balance	Stability
Light	**Slow**	**IB**	
Medium	**Medium**		
Heavy	**Fast**		
	Rhythm		

2. Back lunge

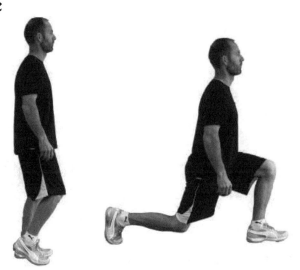

Step backward, starting by bending the front knee while keeping the knee over the foot; the back leg stays loose. Initiate the push up with the front leg.

Resistance	Speed	Balance	Stability
Light	Slow	IB	
Medium	Medium		
Heavy	Fast		
	Rhythm		

KAI FUSSER

3. Front to back lunge

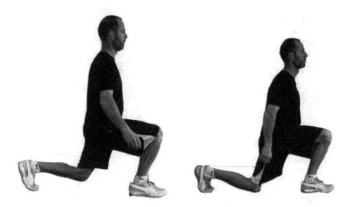

This is a great two for one exercise; very efficient. Combine the front and back lunges by stepping through without stopping, building a good rhythm. If your upper body moves off your axis, you will know that the abs are not engaged.

Resistance	Speed	Balance	Stability
Light	**Slow**	IB	
Medium	**Medium**		
Heavy	**Fast**		
	Rhythm		

4. Front to back lunge on board

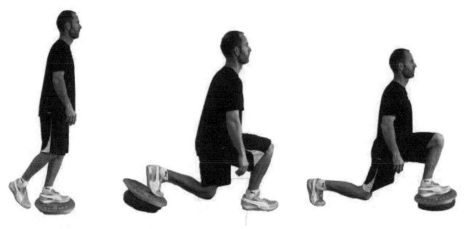

Great for balance, the more you relax the easier it will be.

Resistance	Speed	Balance	Stability
Light	Slow		
Medium	Medium		
	Fast		
	Rhythm		

5. Diagonal lunge

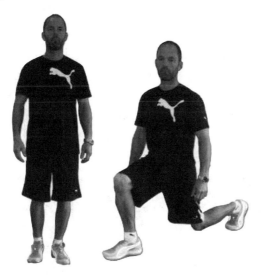

Step out in a 45-degree angle while keeping the upper body facing toward the mirror. Make sure to rotate and align the rear foot with the leg.

Resistance	Speed	Balance	Stability
Light	Slow		
Medium	Medium		
	Rhythm		

6. Plié lunge

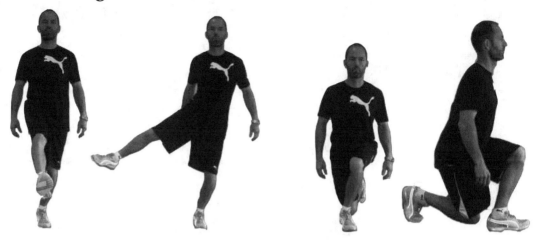

I like this one for the amount of balance and stabilization required of the ankle. Starting with a bent front leg, swing the leg around and squat back with the front leg, keeping the knee over the foot. Sit back into your gluteus as much as possible. Push up off the front leg and swing the leg back to the starting position. Stay relaxed during the whole exercise and feel like you are turning around the center of your body.

Resistance	Speed	Balance	Stability
Light	**Slow**	**IB**	
Medium	**Medium**		
	Rhythm		

7. Plié lunge on board

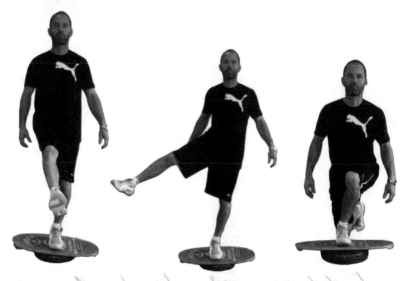

Great for building up the stabilizers in the legs and strengthening balance. The more you relax, the easier this exercise will be. Feel as you turn around the center of your body.

Resistance	Speed	Balance	Stability
Light	Slow		
Medium	Medium		
	Rhythm		

8. Jumping front to back lunge

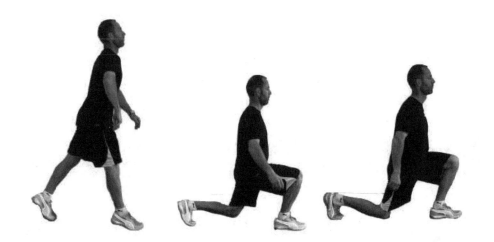

This requires some coordination. Stay relaxed and let your body work for you.

Jump up with the use of your front leg, find a seamless transition and "bounce" back up, as if you are on a trampoline.

Resistance	Speed	Balance	Stability
Light	Slow		
	Medium		
	Fast		
	Rhythm		

9. Twisting, walking lunge

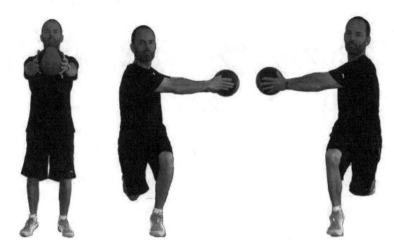

Great for gaining shoulder rotation, coordination and the engagement of the abs. While continuously stepping forward, rotate the shoulders toward the front leg. Keep the arms in front of the shoulders; a 90-degree shoulder turn is ideal. This is best performed by walking toward a mirror to check on your alignment. If your upper body moves off the axis of your lower body, the abs are not engaged and the connection has been lost.

Resistance	Speed	Balance	Stability
Light	**Slow**		
	Medium		
	Rhythm		

10. DB squat

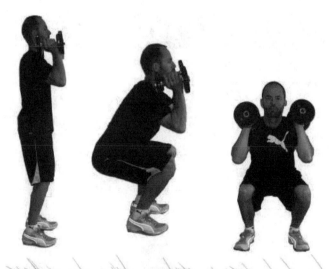

Great exercise to build the gluteus, quadriceps and hamstrings. Hold the DB resting above the elbows, and initiate squat by pushing the hips back; sit on the heels. Initiate the upward movement with the gluteus while drawing in your abs. Your knees should not travel in front of your toes. If you have trouble sitting back, stand in front of a bench and sit back onto it until you touch and return to the top. This will give you the confidence to sit back.

Resistance	Speed	Balance	Stability
Light	Slow	IB	
Medium	Medium		
Heavy	Fast		

11. DB squat on board

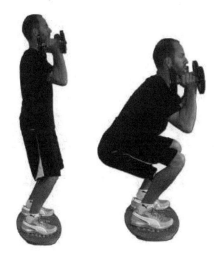

The more you relax, the easier this will be. Let your body move freely.

Resistance	Speed	Balance	Stability
Light	Slow		IB
↓ Heavy			

KAI FUSSER

12. BB squat

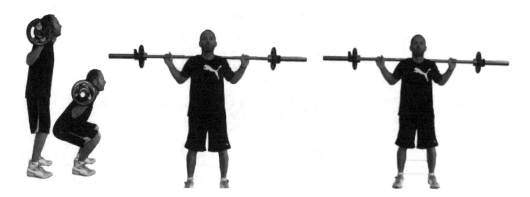

This is one of the big power builders. It requires your whole body to work and builds great strength in the gluteus. Note: your DB squats should be perfect and comfortable before you start with the BB squat. Place the bar onto your shoulders (not the neck), draw your abs in and initiate the squat by moving the hips back. Squat as far as is comfortable but not past the point where your thighs are no longer parallel to the floor. Re-engage the abs and push up with your gluteus. If going heavy, always use a spotter for safety.

Do not place anything under heels and don't look up.

Resistance	Speed	Balance	Stability
Light	Slow		
↓			
Max	Medium		

13. Cable abductor

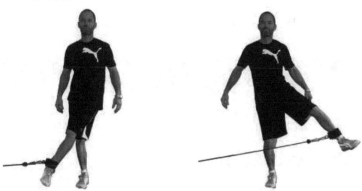

Great exercise for abductor and ankle stabilizer strength building as well as balance. With cable attached to the ankle, let the leg stretch toward the cable. Swing the leg out and away from you through a full range of motion while keep-

WEIGHT TRAINING FOR GOLF

ing the body aligned; return slowly. This should feel like you are turning around the center of your body. Stay relaxed and let your body move.

Resistance	Speed	Balance	Stability
Light	Slow	IB	
	Medium		
	Rhythm		

14. Cable adductor

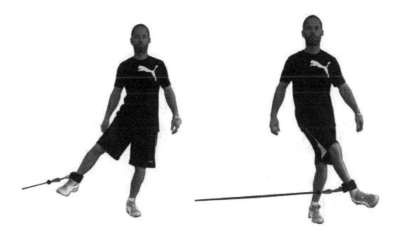

With cable attached to the ankle let the leg be stretched toward the cable, swing leg in to full range of motion while keeping the body aligned. Return slowly and feel like you are turning around the center of your body, stay relaxed and let your body move

Resistance	Speed	Balance	Stability
Light	Slow	IB	
	Medium		
	Rhythm		

15. Cable front extension

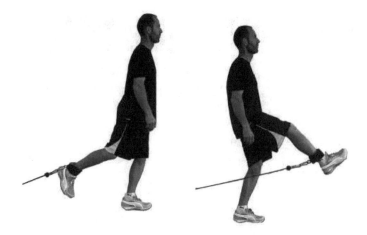

With cable attached to the ankle, face away and let the leg stretch toward the cable. Kick the straight (not locked) leg forward through a full range of motion and return slowly.

Resistance	Speed	Balance	Stability
Light	Slow	IB	
	Medium		
	Rhythm		

16. Cable back extension

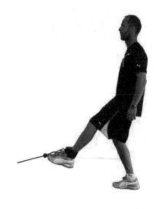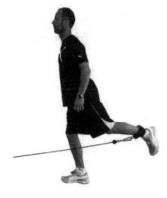

Good exercise to learn to engage the gluteus. With cable attached to the ankle and facing the column, let the leg stretch toward the cable. Kick the straight (not locked) leg backward through a full range of motion. Feel in the back position that the gluteus are engaged. Return slowly.

Resistance	Speed	Balance	Stability
Light	Slow	IB	
	Medium		
	Rhythm		

17. Step up

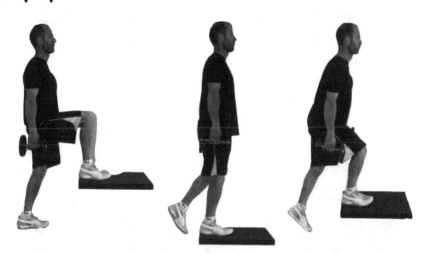

Stand with one foot on the step, making sure that the knee is not extended in front of your foot. Step up by using the front leg. Feel yourself using your gluteus as much as possible. Extend to the top and slowly lower your body back again, feeling how the gluteus controls the speed when you step down.

Resistance	Speed	Balance	Stability
Light	Slow		
Medium	Medium		
Heavy	Rhythm		

CORE

These are all "real" core exercises that have a high carryover to functionality rather than just looks. With each one of them, look to find the connection between your hands and your feet.

1. Crunches on ball

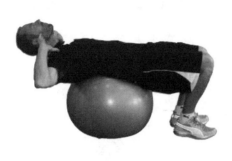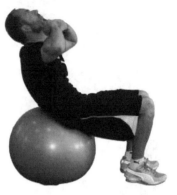

Starting with the small of the back resting on the ball and feet under the knees, draw abs in toward the ball and lift shoulders toward the ceiling without curling the head. Keep looking up toward the ceiling. You can increase the resistance by holding a DB just above your chest.

Resistance	Speed	Balance	Stability
Light	Slow		
↓			
Heavy	Medium		

2. Crunches on ball one leg

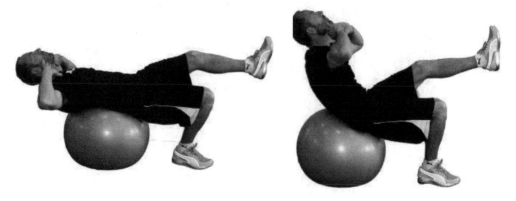

This makes the crunch much harder, as you now have to balance side to side as well.

Resistance	Speed	Balance	Stability
Light	Slow		
Medium	Medium		
Heavy			

3. Superman on ball

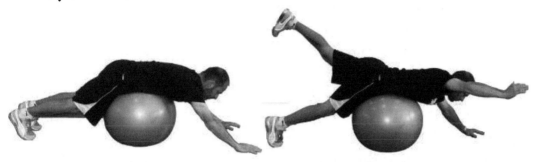

Great for the gluteus and back extensors. Place the ball in the middle of your body, engage the abs and lift opposite arm and leg at the same time. Emphasize to engage the gluteus in the top position.

Resistance	Speed	Balance	Stability
Light	Slow		
	Medium		

KAI FUSSER

WEIGHT TRAINING FOR GOLF

4. Supine hip extension on ball

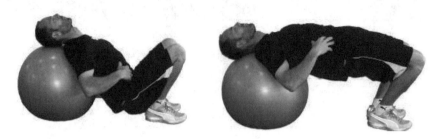

Good exercise for learning to engage the abs and gluteus to connect the upper and lower body into one unit and to produce power through the use of the gluteus and hips. Lie with the upper back and shoulders resting on the ball; the feet should be right under the knees. While almost touching the ground, engage the abs and gluteus and thrust the hips upward to the highest possible position, hold for a couple seconds (feel the abs and gluteus in control) and lower to starting position; repeat. You can place a weight plate onto your hips.

Resistance	Speed	Balance	Stability
Light ↓ **Heavy**	**Slow**		

5. Supine hip extension on ball, one leg

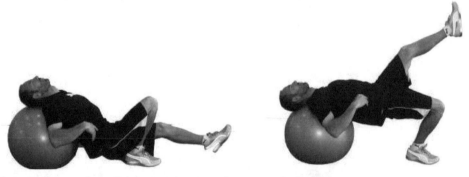

This version makes this exercise much more challenging.

Resistance	Speed	Balance	Stability
Light ↓ **Heavy**	**Slow** **Medium**		

6. Hamstring curl on ball

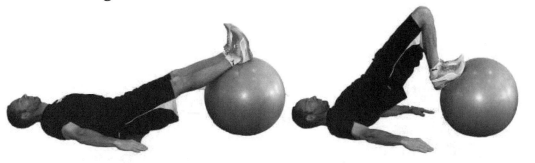

Great hamstring and connection exercise. With your heels on the ball, start by pushing up your hips up to the ceiling and curl the heels in as far as possible. Hold the top position with the abs and gluteus engaged. Make sure your legs are well warmed up for this exercise as it puts quite a strain on your hamstrings.

Resistance	Speed	Balance	Stability
Light	Slow		
	Medium		

7. Hamstring curl on ball, one leg

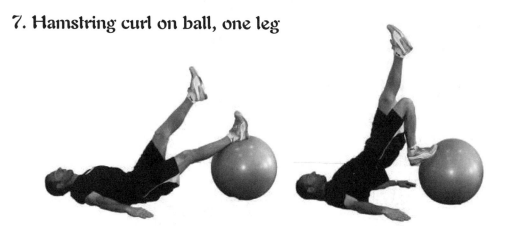

This version makes this exercise much harder. Make sure the legs are well warmed up.

Resistance	Speed	Balance	Stability
Light	Slow		

8. Obliques on ball

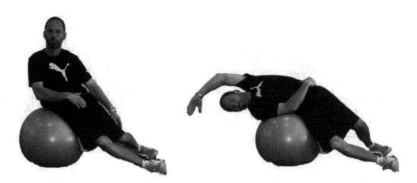

Great exercise for oblique strength and also a great stretch at the same time. Place the side of the hips on the ball, brace the feet against the ground (or against a wall to make it more stable), and lower the upper body sideways as far as it still is comfortable, while also feeling a good stretch (body should stay in line, no bending in the waist). Engage the abs and raise the upper body up and feel as to squeeze the rib cage against the hip bone; slowly lower to the starting position.

Resistance	Speed	Balance	Stability
Light	Slow		
Medium	Medium		

9. Obliques on ball with MB

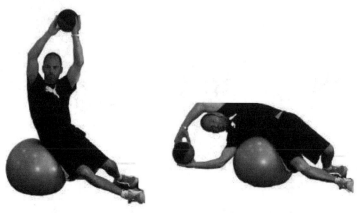

This makes this exercise much harder and also adds more stretch.

Resistance	Speed	Balance	Stability
Light	Slow		
Medium	Medium		

10. Prone jackknife

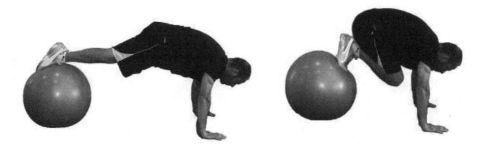

I like this exercise as it really builds a good connection between the hands and the feet. Start in the pushup position with abs drawn toward the ceiling. Pull legs in and tuck knees toward chest, hold for a second and return to starting position.

Resistance	Speed	Balance	Stability
Light	**Slow**		
	Medium		
	Fast		

11. Prone jackknife one leg

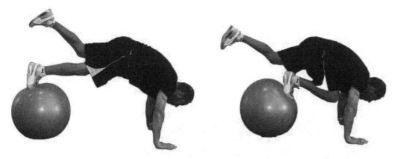

A harder version of this exercise.

Resistance	Speed	Balance	Stability
Light	**Slow**		
	Medium		
	Fast		

12. Supine shoulder rotation on ball

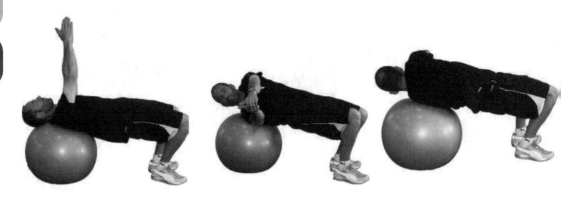

Good exercise to learn to rotate the shoulders and hips by also stabilizing the body through the use of the abs. Lie with the upper back and the shoulders resting on the ball, with the feet directly beneath the knees. Engage the abs and gluteus and push the hips up until they are parallel to the floor. Rotate the shoulders and hips from side to side while maintaining the hips in the upward position. This exercise can also be done with holding a weight or MB with extended arms in front of the chest.

Resistance	Speed	Balance	Stability
Light	**Slow**		
Medium	**Medium**		
	Fast		

13. Plank

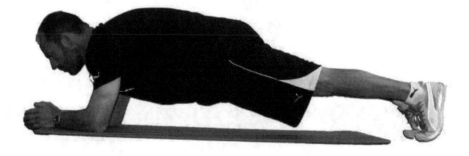

A very popular exercise, great to learn to connect the upper and lower body into one unit. Set up with the toes and elbows on the ground, and then lift the hips up by drawing the abs in. Tilt the hips under and toward the torso while also engaging the gluteus. Looking from the side, the lower back should be slightly rounded upward (no reverse C in the lower back), and the stress should only be felt in the abs and not in the lower back. Hold this posture as long as good form is maintained. If you can hold this position for more than 30 seconds at a time, start taking away stability as seen in 15, 16, 17.

Also, if you are 100% in control of this exercise (through your abs) weight can be added by placing a plate on your upper back.

Resistance	Speed	Balance	Stability
Light	Static		
↓ Heavy			

14. Plank, one leg

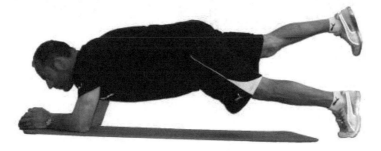

Keep the hips parallel to the floor by control through your core (do not rotate the hips).

Resistance	Speed	Balance	Stability
Light	Static		

15. Plank, one arm

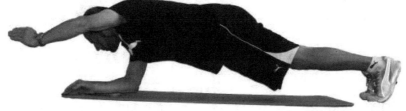

Keep the hips parallel to the floor by control through your core (do not rotate the hips).

Resistance	Speed	Balance	Stability
Light	Static		

16. Plank, one arm, one leg

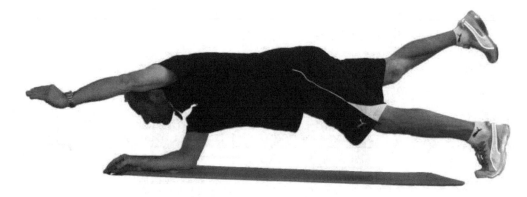

Keep the hips parallel to the floor by control through your core (do not rotate hips).

Resistance	Speed	Balance	Stability
Light	**Static**		

17. Plank, no arms

You may think this is impossible to do, but look at me...we always joke about this in the gym that someday someone will be able to do it.

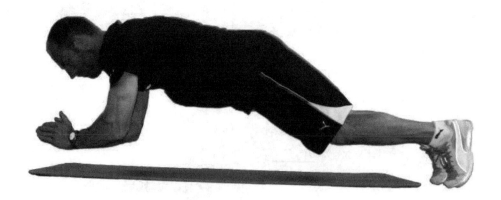

This is a tough one. It took me years to master but I finally did it on April 1, 2011. Once I am able to hold it for longer than 30 seconds, I will try it without legs as well.

18. Side plank on elbow

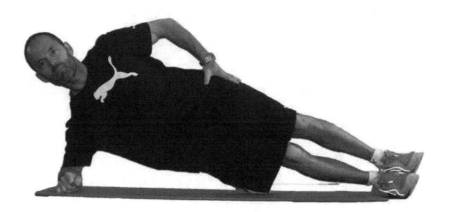

Great oblique and connection exercise. Set up with the feet stacked one on top of the other and the elbow on the ground, Engage the abs and raise the middle of the body off the ground without bending at the waist. Hold for up to 30 seconds, when holding becomes easy, start moving the hips up and down.

Resistance	Speed	Balance	Stability
Light	Static		
	Slow		
	Medium		

KAI FUSSER

19. Side plank on the arm

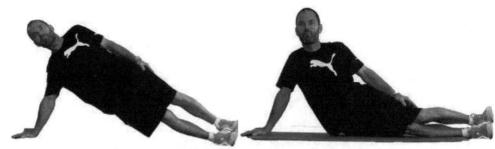

This version requires much more stability from the abs as well as the shoulder.

Set up with the feet stacked one on top of the other and the hand on the ground with a straight (not locked) arm, raise the middle of the body off the ground without bending at the waist. Hold for up to 30 seconds, When holding becomes easy, start moving the hips up and down.

Resistance	Speed	Balance	Stability
Light	Static		IB
	Slow		
	Medium		

20. Hanging abs

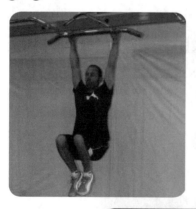
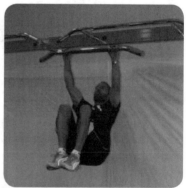
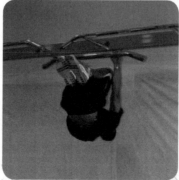

This may be one of the best abdominal exercises there is. It builds the connection between your hands and hips like no other one I know. It is tough but hang in there; it will pay off. (It took Annika two years to be able to curl the hips up all away from a still stand.) Make sure that your shoulders are warmed up well first. Start with and maintain a 90-degree bend between the hips and the thighs (don't just lift your legs). Draw the abs in and rotate hips up as far as possible while also slightly pulling up with your arms. Return slowly to starting position. Even moving only one inch should be considered a success.

Resistance	Speed	Balance	Stability
Light	Static		
	Slow		
	Medium		

21. Pushup hold rotation

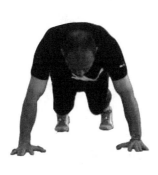 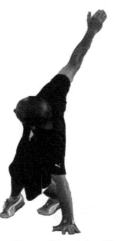

Another good one for connection and stabilization. Start in the pushup position, engage the abs and rotate the shoulders with an extended arm as far as comfortable while keeping the spine neutral. Return slowly to starting position and control the speed of the rotation with the abs. Repeat without putting the rotation hand on the ground.

Resistance	Speed	Balance	Stability
Light	Slow		IB
	Medium		

22. Pushup hold rotation with reach through

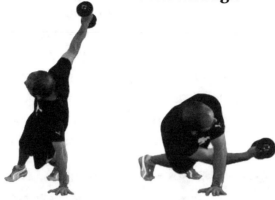

This is the harder version of the pushup hold rotation and requires a lot of core connection strength. Start in the pushup position holding a light DB (2 to 5 pounds). Engage the abs and rotate the shoulders while extending the arm as far as comfortable and keeping the spine neutral. Return slowly past the starting position and reach through with the arm while turning the hips as far as possible, control the speed of the rotation with the abs and repeat without putting the rotation hand on the ground.

Resistance	Speed	Balance	Stability
Light	**Slow**		**IB**
	Medium		

23. Knee to elbow

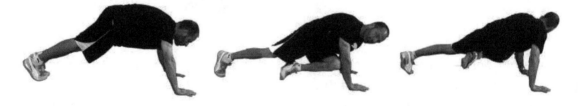

Set up on knees and hands, engage abs and extend the leg all away out while engaging the gluteus in the top position. Draw the knee as close as possible toward the elbow and return back.

Resistance	Speed	Balance	Stability
Light	Slow		IB
	Medium		
	Fast		

24. Ab scissors

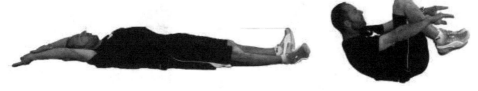

Lying on your back, draw the abs toward the floor. In one swift motion, simultaneously draw the knees and shoulders toward each other and return. Repeat without stopping.

Resistance	Speed	Balance	Stability
Light	Slow		
	Medium		
	Fast		

ROTATIONAL

Rotational exercises are great for full body engagement and for learning to load and unload the body just like you want to do in the swing. They also represent many parts of the swing, which helps teach the body the right movement patterns.

1. One arm cable push

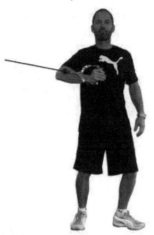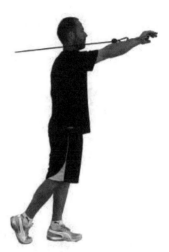

Great to initiate the rotation and create power with your legs and hips. Finish in a complete and balanced position stacked over your left leg, with hips pointing toward the "target." Set up with your axis intact and hips in line with the cable, relax arm and grip, knees slightly bent.

Start by engaging the abs, initiating the rotation from the ground up: legs, hips, torso, shoulders, and then arm. Complete the finish with the hips pointing to the target, back leg extended with gluteus engaged; upper body stacked over the straight, not locked, front leg; and feeling the weight transfer from the back leg to the front leg. Avoid falling into a reverse C by keeping the abs engaged. Return slowly, by controlling the return speed with your abs.

Resistance	Speed	Balance	Stability
Light	**Slow**		
Medium	**Medium**		
Heavy	**Fast**		
	Rhythm		

WEIGHT TRAINING FOR GOLF

2. One arm cable pull

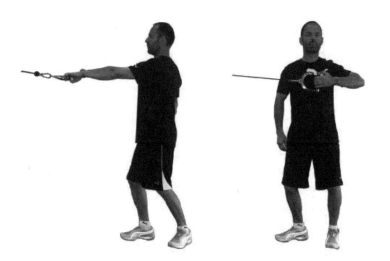

Great for rotating the body together while maintaining the axis, leading with the hips and not pulling with the arm. Set up with your axis intact, with hips perpendicular to the cable. Relax arm and grip with knees slightly bent. Start by engaging your abs and then initiate the rotation with the hips. The upper body and arm will follow, just slightly delayed. Feel as the whole body works as one unit. The hand and arm should end up in line with the cable without any kinks. Finish with a solid and balanced stance still within your axis; return slowly with the abs controlling the speed.

KAI FUSSER

Resistance	Speed	Balance	Stability
Light	**Slow**		
Medium	**Medium**		
Heavy	**Fast**		
	Rhythm		

WEIGHT TRAINING FOR GOLF

3. Straight cable rotation

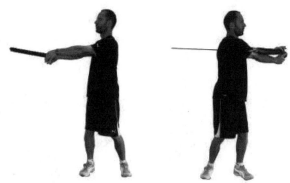

One of the best rotational exercises to learn to rotate around a straight axis, keeping the connection between the arms and the shoulders, and to load and unload the body. Set up with a straight axis, holding the rope with a loose grip and extending (not locking) arms in front of the shoulders (the created triangle between the arms and shoulders stays intact). Engage the abs and rotate the shoulders about 90 degrees and hips about 50 degrees to the back side while sitting into your back leg. Re-engage the abs and rotate to the front, starting from the ground up with legs-hips-torso-shoulders-arms while keeping a perfect axis. Finish with shoulders at 90 degrees to the cable. There should be a slight weight shift from the back leg to the front leg. Return slowly with the abs controlling the speed.

Resistance	Speed	Balance	Stability
Light	**Slow**		
Medium	**Medium**		
Heavy	**Fast**		
	Rhythm		

4. Wood chop down

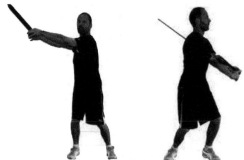

Another great exercise for rotational power and control. Have the shoulders face the cable with extended arms (not locked). Keep the triangle between the arms and shoulders intact. With a loose grip engage the abs and initiate the rotation with the hips followed by the shoulders and arms, sit down slightly and complete the rotation to shoulders being square to the cable and return slowly with the abs controlling the speed.

Resistance	Speed	Balance	Stability
Light	Slow		IB
Medium	Medium		
Heavy	Fast		
	Rhythm		

5. Wood chop up

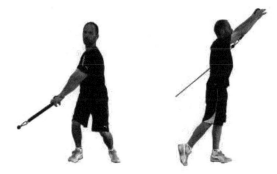

This is one of my favorites, it requires the whole body to work together and build great core strength. If you would only have 10 minutes to work out I would do this exercise, 3-5 sets of 8 reps.

Have the shoulders face the cable with extended arms (not locked), keep the triangle between the arms and shoulders intact. Sit into your back leg with a loose grip and engage the abs. Initiate upward rotation from bottom up, starting with leg, then hip, shoulders, and arms. Get into a good finish position with full rotation, shoulders over hips and ankle and full extension (avoid a reverse C). Feel the weight transfer from the back to the front leg. Lower the rope slowly with arms extended and with shoulders relaxed, making sure that the abs protect the back and control the speed.

Resistance	Speed	Balance	Stability
Light	Slow		IB
Medium	Medium		
Heavy	Fast		
	Rhythm		

KAI FUSSER

With these power exercises you will learn to create and release all available power in an instant. Some can also be performed at about the same rhythm as your swing, so you can practice re-engaging your abs just before the change of direction, which will connect your upper and lower bodies for good energy transfer and control.

1. Power clean

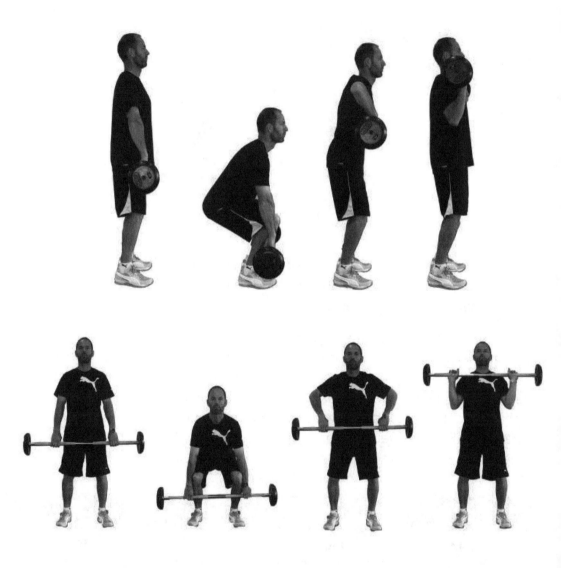

This is one of the best power exercises there is. It requires the whole body to work together. Start easy on this and learn it to perfection. I recommend that you seek the help of a trainer when learning this exercise as you could injure yourself when performed incorrectly.

Start with a loose grip just wider than the hips, engage the abs and sit back. With a neutral spine, lean forward enough so the bar will clear the hips, and start the upward movement by engaging the abs again. Drive from the ground up, using the gluteus and your lats to pull the bar up in a explosive motion. Maintain a loose grip throughout and keep the bar as close as possible to your body. You should feel yourself becoming "free" of the bar after it passes your midsection. Then, tuck your elbows in and let the bar come down into your hands and sit into your legs. To get back to the starting position, engage the abs and "toss" the bar upward while keeping it close to your body. When free of the bar, bring the elbows up and lower it. You should never feel that you are "lifting" the bar or that the bar comes away from you.

Resistance	Speed	Balance	Stability
Light	Medium		
Medium	Fast		
Heavy	Rhythm		

KAI FUSSER

2. Dead lift

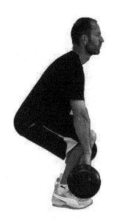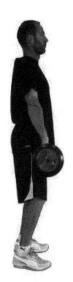

This is basically a half-power clean, great for learning to build power from the ground up. Start with a loose grip just wider then the hips, engage the abs and sit back. With a neutral spine, lean forward enough so the bar will clear the knees. Start the upward movement by engaging the abs again, driving from the ground up, using the gluteus to the straight position with the shoulders back and chest up.

Resistance	Speed	Balance	Stability
Light	Medium		
Medium	Fast		
Heavy	Rhythm		

WEIGHT TRAINING FOR GOLF

3. Shot put

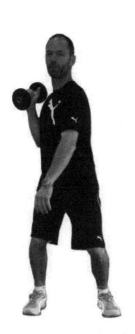 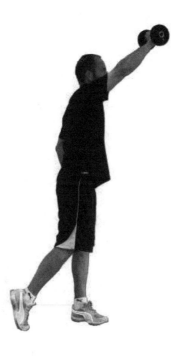

Set up in a shot put position, sitting into the back leg to load it up while maintaining your axis. Engage the abs and initiate the acceleration and rotation from the ground up — legs, hips, torso, shoulders, and then arm. Rotate to a full finish with the hips pointing toward the target, legs, upper body and arm extended. Be balanced and stacked over the straight but not locked front leg (avoid a reverse C by keeping the abs engaged; do not lock the knee).

Resistance	Speed	Balance	Stability
Light	Medium		
Medium	Fast		
Heavy	Rhythm		

KAI FUSSER

4. MB throw to wall

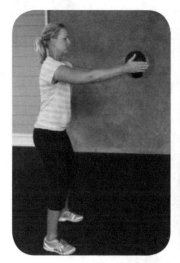 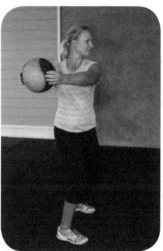

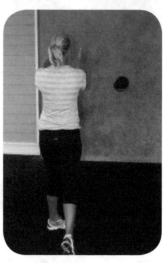

Set up with a straight axis, holding the ball with a loose grip and extended (not locked) arms in front of the shoulders (the created triangle between the arms and shoulders stays intact). Engage the abs and rotate the shoulders about 90 degrees and hips about 50 degrees to the back side. Re-engage the abs and rotate to the front, starting from the ground up, starting with legs, then hips, torso, shoulders and finally arms, while keeping a perfect axis. There should be a seamless transition at the change of direction. Release the ball at the apex of the rotation; the hands should not "throw" the ball. Finish with the hips and shoulders pointing towards target in a balanced finish position and feel the weight transfer from the back leg to the front leg. Avoid a reverse C by keeping the abs engaged; do not lock the knees.

Resistance	Speed	Balance	Stability
Light	Slow		
Medium	Medium		
	Rhythm		

5. MB throw sitting

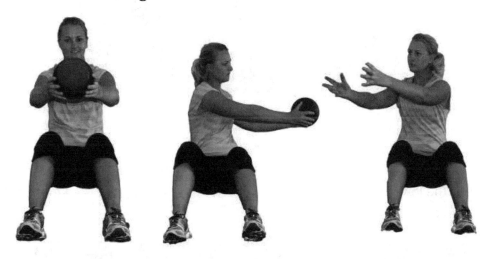

This is all about the core and shoulder rotation as the hips and legs are isolated and can't assist. This is a great exercise to learn to connect the shoulders to the midsection.

Have a partner throw the ball to you. Engage the abs before you touch the ball and keep the arms out in front of your chest (keep the triangle intact) and let the force of the ball turn your upper body. Just before the turn around, re-engage your abs and rotate the shoulders forward. Release the ball from your hands at the apex of the rotation, back toward your partner. You should feel that it is the rotation of the upper body that accelerates the ball and not your arms throwing it.

Resistance	Speed	Balance	Stability
Light	Slow		
Medium	Medium		
	Rhythm		

6. MB slam

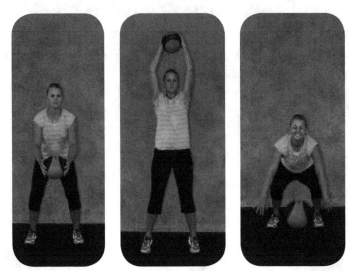

This is fun. Go all out and learn how to release all your power in an instant. Set up with straight (not locked) arms, engage the abs and accelerate from the ground up to the fully extended top position. Just before the turn around, re-engage the abs and slam the ball to the ground by drawing your upper body toward the lower body at full speed. Make sure there is a good transition at the top turn around without stopping.

Resistance	Speed	Balance	Stability
Light	**Medium**		
Medium	**High**		

7. Bench jump

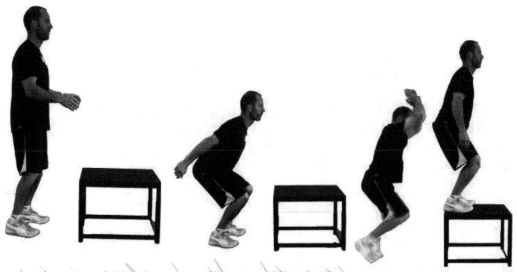

This is another great exercise to learn to release your power with one quick move. Start with a low stepper as the height itself is not critical; however, how high you jump is. In the upright starting position, squat down and engage your abs just before the turn around. In an explosive motion from the ground up, accelerate to the top and into the jump, swing the relaxed arms in coordination with the jump to increase the energy released. Land on the bench with soft legs and step back (not jump) down to the floor to start over.

Resistance	Speed	Balance	Stability
Light	Medium		
Medium	High		

8. Get ups

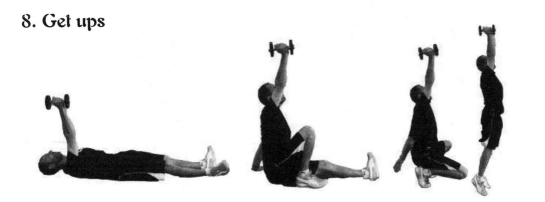

This is a tough one and will require power combined with coordination. It also works great for high intensity interval training.

Lie flat on the ground and hold one arm up toward the ceiling. Draw the abs in and accelerate the upper body and legs up to the get up position. With the help of the opposite arm, push off the ground and jump as high as possible, with full extension. The raised arm should point toward the ceiling throughout the exercise. Lower yourself down to the starting position while keeping your abs engaged. Try to create a good rhythm without stopping. Do four to eight reps and then switch to other side.

Resistance	Speed	Balance	Stability
Light	Slow		
	Medium		
	High		

WEIGHT TRAINING FOR GOLF

9. Pushup to jump

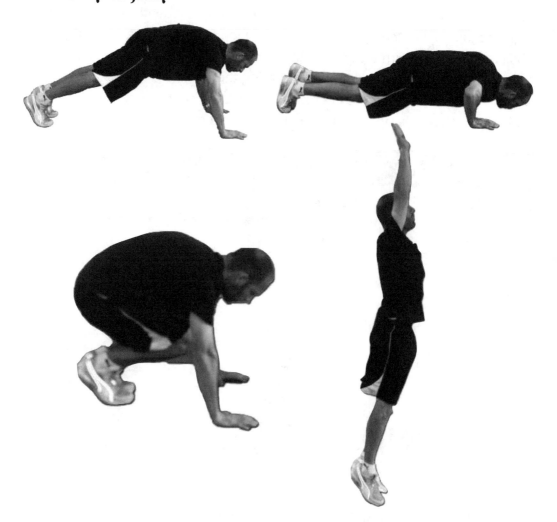

This is very similar to the get ups and involves your whole body. Also great for high intensity interval training. Starting in the pushup position, lower the body and, by drawing the abs up toward the ceiling, accelerate up and pull the knees in under you. Push up with the legs and jump to a fully extended position using the swinging of your arms for momentum, and quickly come back down to the pushup position, making sure the abs are engaged to protect your back. Do four to eight repetitions with good rhythm.

Resistance	Speed	Balance	Stability
Light	**Slow**		
	Medium		
	High		

A couple Challenges:

One arm one leg pushup

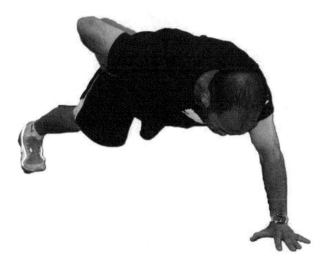

This is tough and requires extreme core strength in order to connect your hand to your foot. Try holding it first without movement, when comfortable start moving down little by little.

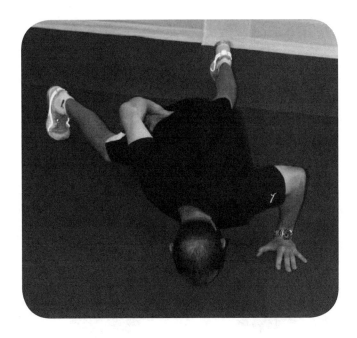

Two ball pushup with two feet

A fun challenge which requires tremendous core and balance control as both balls want to move into all directions.

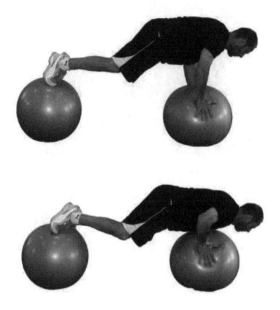

Two ball pushup with one foot

This is the real deal, do 8 reps and send me video of it !

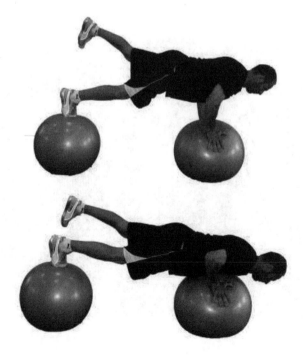

RUBBER BAND

Most cable and some dumbbell exercises can be performed using a rubber band instead. I still prefer the cable or dumbbell for strength building, however. The advantage of using the rubber band is that you can take advantage of its springiness when doing exercises with rhythm or at full speed. Also, you can take a rubber band with you anywhere you go and keep up on the exercises.

The exercises are performed the same way as with a cable or dumbbell. Adjust the resistance by using different strength bands or by shortening it. Here are just some examples:

1. RB chest press

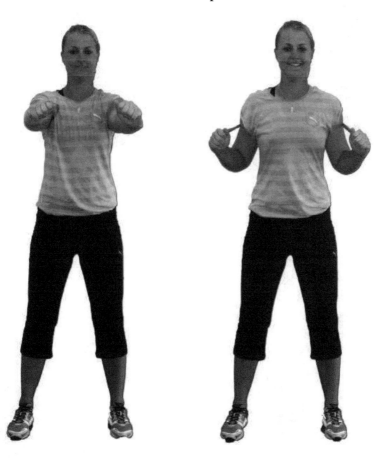

2. RB push

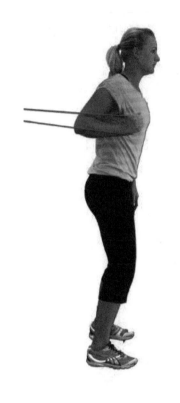
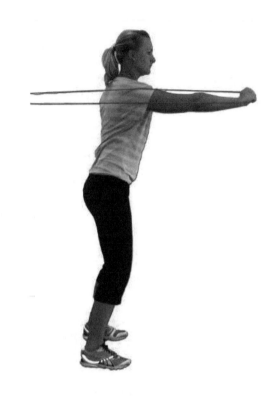

3. RB pull

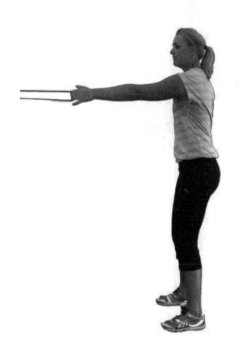
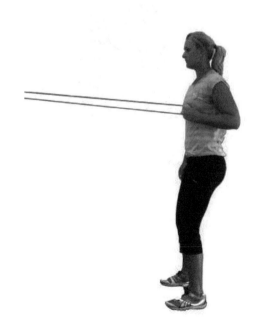

4. RB twisting curl to over head

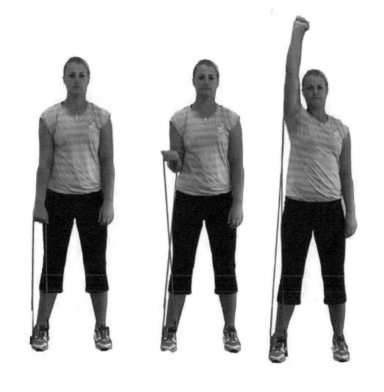

5. RB triceps kick back

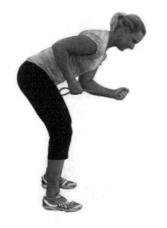 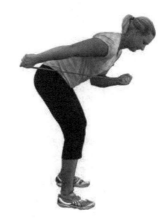

6. RB shot put

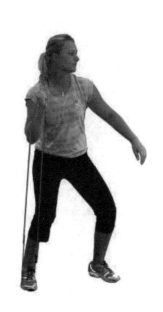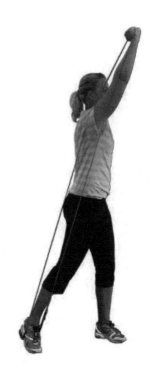

7. RB straight rotation

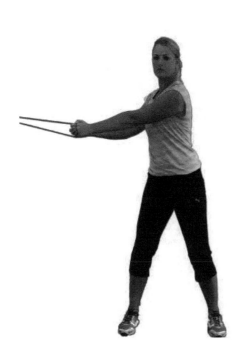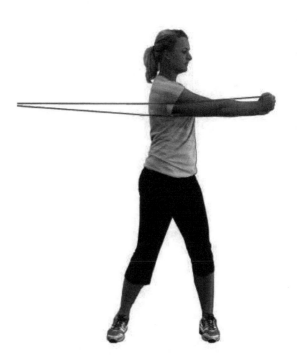

STRETCHES

1. Iliopsoas on bench

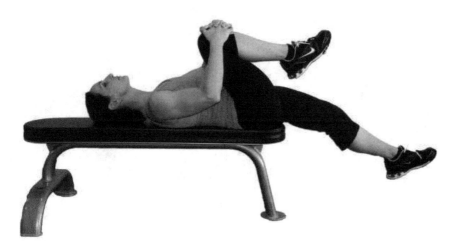

Lie on the bench with your hips right on the edge. Pull the knee toward your chest and hold it. Let the stretching leg relax and you will feel it lower more and more.

2. Hamstring lying

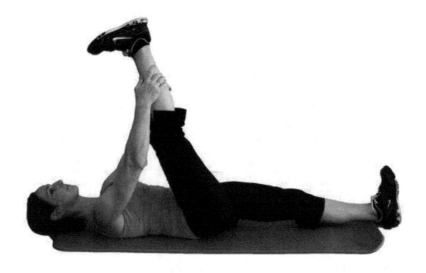

Lie on your back and raise one leg, keeping the other on the ground. Use your hands to pull the raised straight leg toward your chest. You can also use a towel or rubber band around your foot to pull the leg back

3. Gluteus on ball

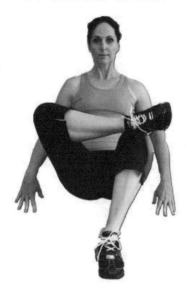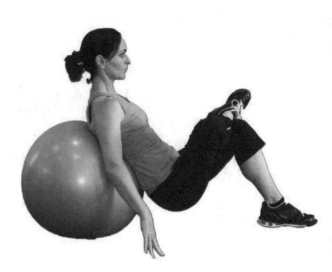

Sit on ball and cross one leg over. Slide down on the ball slowly to a comfortable stretch

4. Gluteus sitting

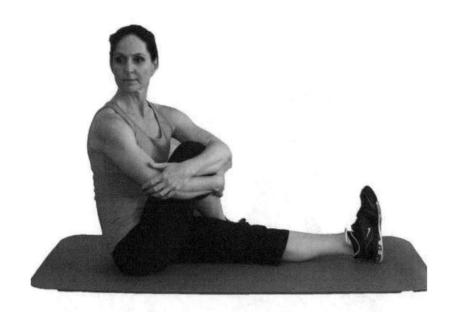

In the sitting position, cross one leg over. Wrap your opposite arm around the knee and pull the leg with your arm to a good stretch. You can rotate your upper body against the leg to add intensity.

5. Quadriceps lying

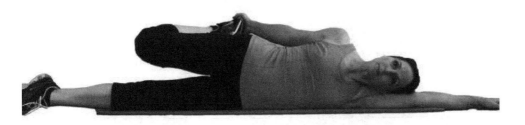

Lie on your side and pull your foot back with your hand until the desired stretch is felt in the quadriceps and also hip flexors.

6. Piriformis

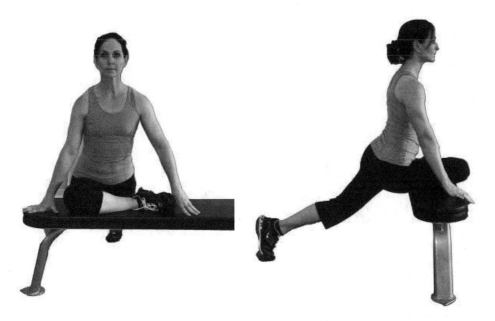

Fold the leg onto the bench and lower the body slowly to a good stretch, using your arms to support your weight as necessary.

KAI FUSSER

7. Ab stretch on ball

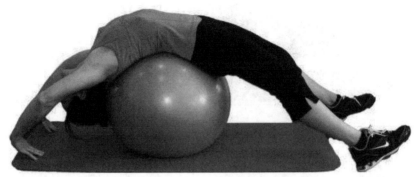

Lie with your shoulders on the ball and slowly push yourself back until you feel a good stretch.

8. Prone cobra elbow

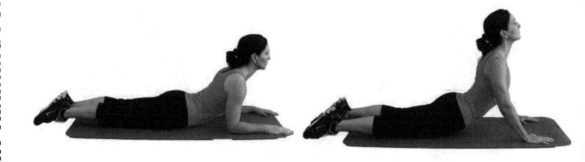

Lying face down on the floor, push your upper body upward with your elbows. (A more advanced version would be using your hands instead of your elbows.) Feel the stretch in your abs.

WEIGHT TRAINING FOR GOLF

9. Spinal rotation RB

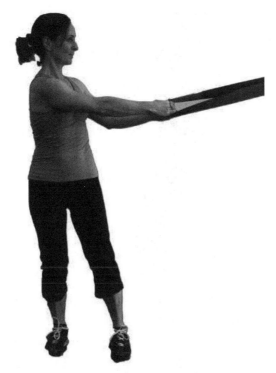

Stand sideways to the rubber band and hold it with your extended arms. Rotate your hips and shoulders against the rubber band. You can also use your body weight to "fall" against the band.

KAI FUSSER

10. Chest and shoulder and biceps RB

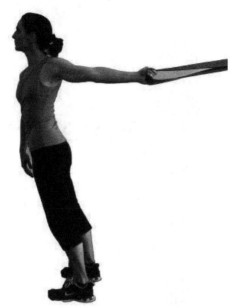

Great stretch for the arms, shoulders and chest area. With a straight and re-laxed arm, let your body weight lean into the rubber band. Rotating the upper body or the arm and hand will give you a stretch in different parts of the body. See which area "feels" good and hold for 45 to 60 seconds and move to the next desired area to stretch. This stretch can also be done with both arms reaching back.

11. Latissimus and back one and two-arm RB

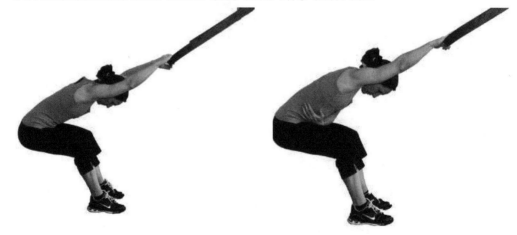

With these two positions you can perform multiple stretches. Keep your grip and arms relaxed and let your body weight help with the stretch. As you rotate the shoulders and upper body, you will feel different areas being stretched.

12. Calf FR

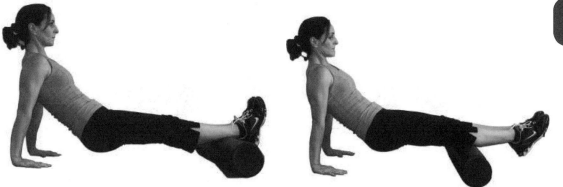

Start by positioning your legs so that the roller is sitting just above the Achilles tendon. With help from your upper body, roll the calves slowly down to just below your knee; go back and forth. You can rotate the legs slightly to address different areas of the calves. Crossing one leg over the other will increase the pressure if needed.

13. Quadriceps FR

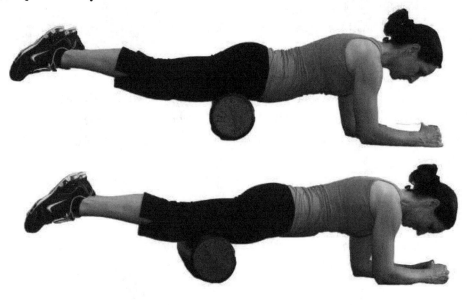

With the upper body supported by the elbows, position your legs so that the roller is just above the knees. Roll down the roller to just below the hips. Here, too, you can rotate the legs slightly to address different areas. Crossing one leg over the other will increase the pressure, if needed.

14. Hamstring FR

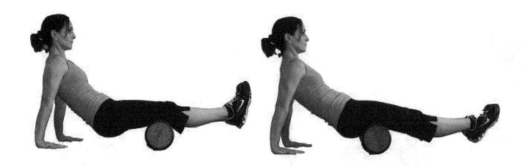

With the upper body supported by the arms, position your legs on the roller just above the knees. Roll down the roller to just below the gluteus. Here, too, you can rotate the legs slightly to address different areas. Crossing one leg over the other will increase the pressure, if needed.

15. IT band FR

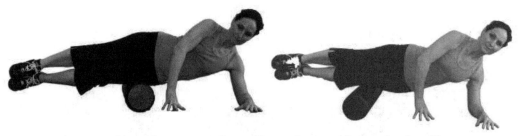

This is a fun one. Lie sideways on the roller and support your body with your arms, starting with the roller just below the hips. Roll down to just above the knee. If the pressure is too much, put the foot of the top leg on the ground to relieve some of the pressure.

16. Gluteus FR

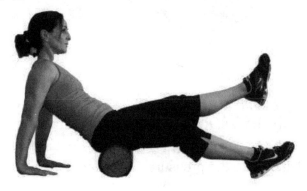

Start by sitting on the roller, supporting your body with your arms. Roll up and down the gluteus while also adding some rotations. Lift up one leg if more pressure is desired.

17. Upper back

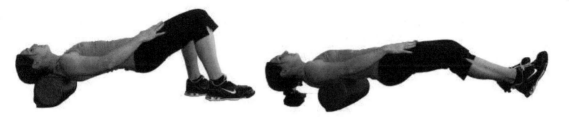

Lie with your upper back on the roller and push your hips off the ground. Roll up on the roller to about the middle of your back.

Swing Fault Exercises

SINCE OPENING THE ANNIKA Academy over four years ago, we have had hundreds of golfers go through our programs, from total beginners to single digit handicappers on up to professionals. Working together so closely as a team, our coaches, Henri Reis, Charlotta Sorenstam and Mark Bereza, with me as the fitness coach, have gathered a lot of experience. Having the practice range, hitting booths with all the video and analysis systems and the gym all under one roof is an invaluable asset. We can communicate and coordinate the needs of our students right there and then, which leads to quick solutions to help the players improve their game.

Out of that experience, we have developed Swing Fault Drills (using the club) and Swing Fault Exercises (performed in the gym). The combination of the two have been very effective.

What we see is that almost all of the swing faults are movement faults that also show up when doing exercises in the gym. For example, when a player doesn't start the down swing with the hips, he also doesn't start the rotational exercises with his hips. When a player doesn't rotate the shoulders during the swing, he also doesn't turn his shoulders during rotational exercises. And, when a player tightens his grip during the swing, he will also tighten the grip during exercising.

Many of these movement faults have developed over the years — the way you stand, walk, bend, jump, turn, lift, push, pull, accelerate, decelerate and so on. The good news is that they can be quickly identified and then fixed. It will take some effort and work, but you are not afraid of that.

The good news is that, once you know your swing faults, you can pick the according swing fault exercises and accelerate your learning process. I would venture to say that one repetition of a perfectly executed swing fault exercise may be worth 50 practice swings on the range. When you are on the range hitting balls and practicing, the feedback is very minimal. It is mainly the ball flight that will reveal to you what went wrong, but that may not be so accurate. It is very hard to really feel where your hips or shoulders are, because at that moment you are occupied by making sure that you hit the ball. That preoccupation slows down the learning process.

Everyone knows what effect the ball can have on your mind. Just compare your practice swing with your real swing. Simply stepping forward those four inches, so much can change. It's that pesky ball that can have that effect on your mind.

Conversely, when you perform a swing fault exercise in the gym, the circumstances are much more conducive to learning. You can take your time, go slowly, watch yourself in the mirror, load up your body with some resistance which will give you greater feedback (you can actually feel which muscles initiate or decelerate a movement) and you don't have to deal with that little ball. That's why these swing fault exercises are so efficient.

They are also great for warm up and preparation before practice or play. Select a couple before hitting balls, depending on what's going on in your swing. Let's say that you feel you are not getting into a complete finish position. You then should do some "shot put" and "one arm push" drills. These will remind your body and help set up your nervous system for the right movement pattern. Even during play, before a shot, you could call on one of these exercises to set your body up for the right movement, right on the tee box (yet with no equipment).

Also realize that every exercise in this book represents some part, no matter how small, of the swing. Combining these exercises results in something very close to the swing movement.

Even if you only do these swing fault exercises and nothing else from this book (not that you would ...) you will see some good results in your game.

Here are the top swing fault exercises. They can be performed in the gym, at home or on the range, with different equipment, including the cable, rubber band, medicine ball, etc.

Keep the resistance low and do as many reps as needed to learn the movement just like you would when practicing your swing. Try to use the mirror as much as possible to correct your form and ingrain a good picture in your mind.

Even though these are specific exercises designed to improve swing, you should always practice them from both sides. The golf swing is one sided enough as it is.

1. Abs in for address position

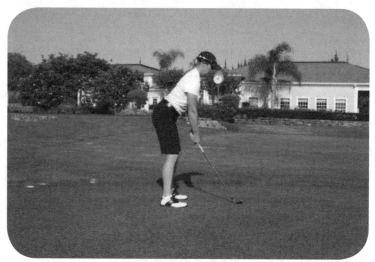

Abs not engaged

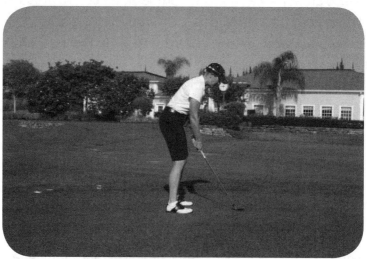

Engaged with slight hip tilt

Purpose: To learn to engage your abs in your address position while maintaining your setup to the ball.

Get into your address position in front of the mirror with the side view. While maintaining your setup, draw the abs in (belly button in) and slightly tilt your hips up toward your head (your belt buckle should tilt more upward). You should also feel that your gluteus is slightly engaged. Looking into the mirror,

WEIGHT TRAINING FOR GOLF

you should see that your lower spine is straight, without a "C" in any direction. Learn to relax the rest of your body and your breathing, so that only your mid-section is engaged. Practice holding and re-engaging this position until it feels normal and comfortable. As a further step, hold that engagement and rotate your shoulders and swing your relaxed arms in a pendulum motion.

2. DB pendulum swing

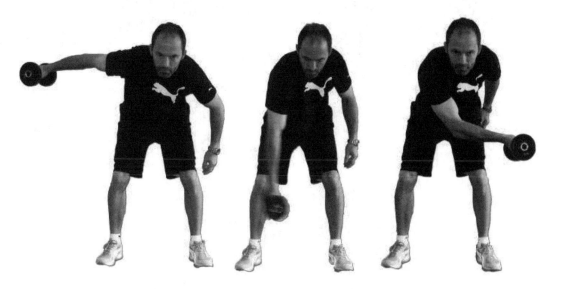

Purpose: To learn to stay relaxed in your arms and grip, learning to use your arms as leverage.

This is also a progression from the "abs in for the address position" exercise.

Stand in your address position with some more upper body forward lean and hold the DB (3 to 5 lbs.) with a very loose grip just in your fingers. Relax your arm and shoulders completely, engage your abs and swing the arm in a pendulum motion, maintaining your spine angle. Feel how much speed you can create in the DB without any effort by staying relaxed. Tightening your grip, arm or shoulder will reveal just how much more energy you must create, and how much more stress there is on your body to recreate that same speed. After some repetitions with the right arm seamlessly switch to the left arm, after that hold the DB with both hands and try to maintain the pendulum effect.

3. Arm connection rotation with club

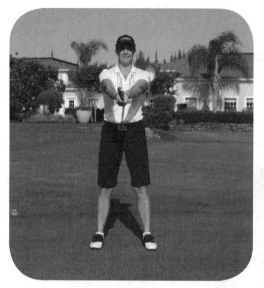 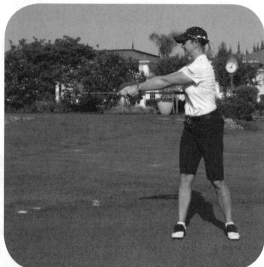

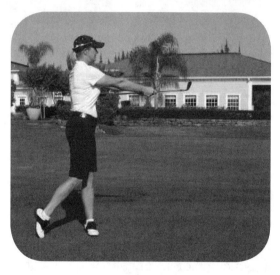

Purpose: To learn to connect your arms to your shoulders, creating a triangle; to learn to rotate your shoulders while maintaining the connection.

Using a stick or golf club, place one end in the middle of your chest and extend your arms fully, Engage your abs and rotate the shoulders about 90 degrees and your hips about 50 degrees. Feel how your arms stay connected to the shoulders. Initiate the forward rotation by rotating your hips with the shoulders and arms following into a good finish position, with the hips facing the target.

4. Back swing cable rotation

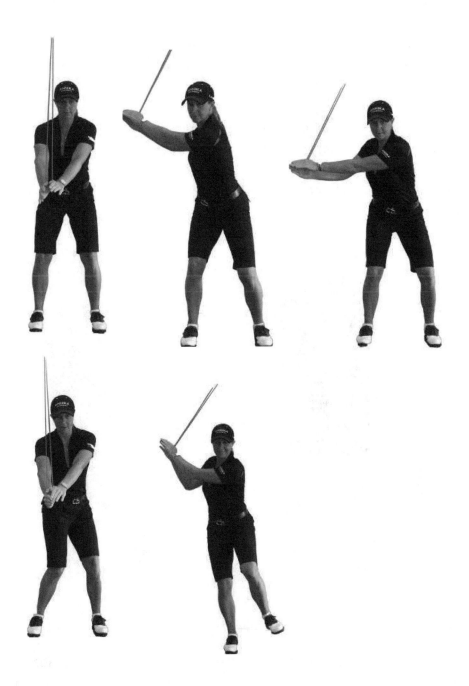

Purpose: To learn to rotate shoulders and arms as one unit without reaching for or losing the connection between your arms and the shoulders, and learn to initiate the down swing rotation from the ground up, starting with the hips.

Set up in a close to address position with arms extended (not locked) right in front of your chest, (the created triangle between the arms and shoulders stays intact). Engage the abs and rotate the shoulders and arms as one unit to about a 90-degree shoulder turn. Your hips should turn about 50 degrees. Feel the connection running from your hands through the arms, shoulders, torso, hips and legs. Re-engage the abs and initiate the downswing from the ground up, starting with the legs and hips, and followed by the torso, shoulders and arms. The spine angle, front and side, should be maintained throughout this exercise. The rubber band may also be used here.

5. Cable hip rotation rope

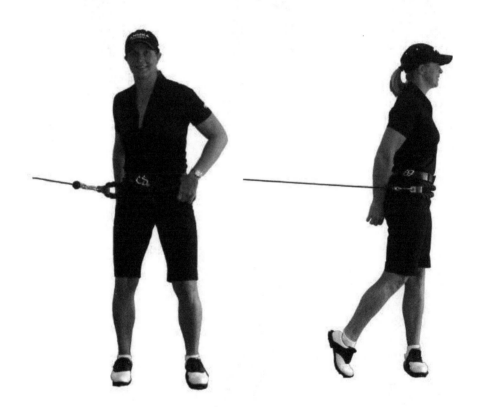

Purpose: To learn to initiate and follow through the rotation with legs and hips.

Set up with the cable/rope held against the hips, engage the abs and initiate the rotation with the hips. Feel the outside (left) of the hip pulling and the inside (right) of the hip pushing to initiate the rotation. Get into a full finish position with the back leg extended, gluteus engaged, stacked over the straight but not locked front leg. The rubber band may also be used here.

6. RB Straight rotation

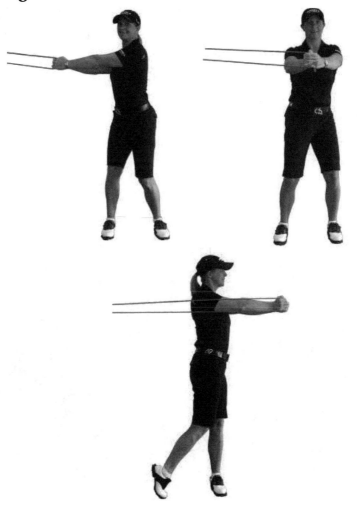

Purpose: To learn to rotate around your axis without leaning or sliding the hips, while keeping your arms and shoulders connected. This exercise is great if you tend to "slide" your hips during the swing.

Set up holding the rope with a loose grip with your arms extended (not locked), creating a triangle between the arms and the shoulders (this triangle stays intact throughout the exercise). Rotate the shoulders about 90 degrees and the hips about 50 degrees toward the cable to the starting position, sitting on top of the inside leg. Engage the abs and initiate the rotation with the hips. Feel the outside (left) of the hip pulling and the inside (right) of the hip pushing to initiate the rotation. The hips should be slightly leading the torso and shoulder-arm connection. Follow the rotation, rotating the shoulders about 90 degrees until they are perpendicular to the cable. The hips should not slide horizontally away from your shoulders or legs.

Throughout this exercise, the axis should stay intact, with the shoulders over the hips, which are over the feet. You should feel a slight weight transfer from the right leg to the left as the whole axis shifts, just like in the swing. Re-engage the abs and slowly rotate back to the starting position. Feel how the abs control the speed of the rotation. Start this exercise slowly until you can do it perfectly, and then try to create the same speed and rhythm as in your swing. Feel how the engagement of the abs just before the turnaround of the rotation (down swing) connects your upper body to your lower body. This exercise can also be done with the cable.

7. MB Straight rotation

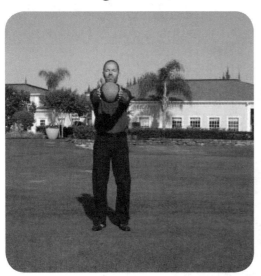
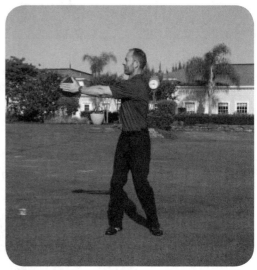
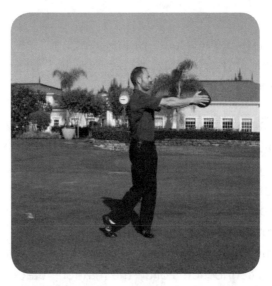

Purpose: To learn to rotate around a straight axis, keeping the connection between the arms and the shoulders; to learn to load and unload the body.

Set up with a straight axis, holding the ball with a loose grip, using extended (not locked) arms in front of the shoulders (the created triangle between the arms and shoulders stays intact). Engage the abs and rotate the shoulders about 90 degrees and the hips about 50 degrees to the back side while sitting into your back leg. Re-engage the abs just before the turnaround and rotate to the front, starting from the ground up with first legs, then hips, torso, shoulders and finally arms, while keeping a perfect axis. There should be a seamless transition at the change of direction without stopping. Get into a full finish position with the hips pointing toward the target with the back leg extended, gluteus engaged, stacked over the straight — not locked — front leg. Feel the weight transfer from the back leg to the front leg. Start this exercise slowly until you can execute it perfectly, and then try to create the same speed and rhythm as in your swing. Feel how the engagement of the abs just before the turnaround of the rotation (down swing) connects your upper body to your lower body.

KAI FUSSER

8. MB throw to wall

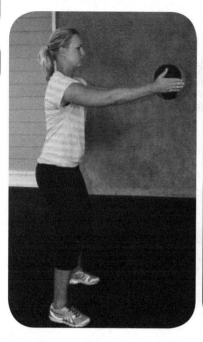 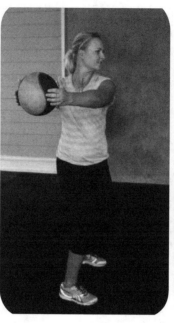 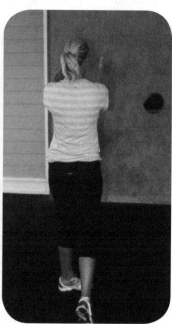

Purpose: To learn to rotate around the axis, maintaining the shoulder-arm connection (triangle); learn to load and unload the body and release the ball with a complete and balanced finish. This is basically the same exercise as the Medicine Ball Rotation, but in this instance, you release the ball.

Set up with a straight axis holding the ball with a loose grip and extended but not locked arms in front of the shoulders (the created triangle between the arms and shoulders stays intact). Engage the abs and rotate the shoulders about 90 degrees and the hips about 50 degrees to the back side. Re-engage the abs and rotate to the front, starting from the ground up beginning with the legs, then hips, torso, shoulders and then arms, while keeping a perfect axis. There should be a seamless transition at the change of direction. Release the ball at the apex of the rotation. The hands should not be used to throw the ball. Finish with the hips pointing toward the target in a balanced finish position, feeling your weight transfer from your back leg to the front leg. Avoid a reverse C by keeping the abs engaged; do not lock the knee.

Start with a four-pound ball. Keep in mind that, the lighter the ball (e.g., a volleyball), the harder this exercise will be, as there is less feedback and the tendency to "throw" or "push" the ball increases.

9. MB Lunge rotation MB

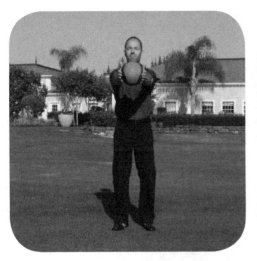 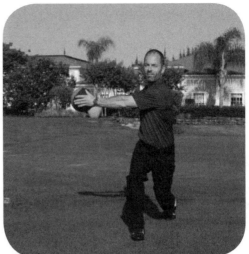

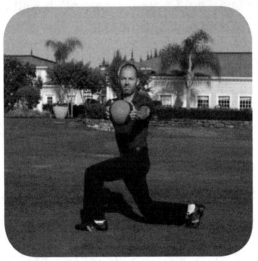

Purpose: To increase the range of motion for torso and shoulder rotation, and increase balance during rotation with the help of the abs connecting the upper and lower body.

Set up with a straight axis, holding the ball with a loose grip and extended — not locked — arms in front of the shoulders (the created triangle between the arms and shoulders stays intact). Engage the abs and step into a lunge. With the abs still engaged, rotate the shoulders to the same side as your forward leg while maintaining the axis. Push back into the starting position and repeat with other leg. When you see that your upper body moves left or right on top of your hips, you'll know that you've lost the connection; control that with your abs. This exercise can be done in a stationary position as well, repeating on the same leg without lunging up, or walking, alternating from one leg to the other, which requires greater balance and coordination.

10. MB Wood chop up

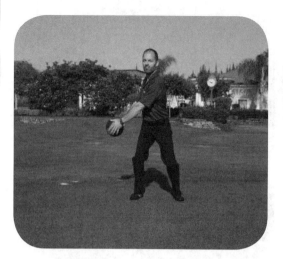 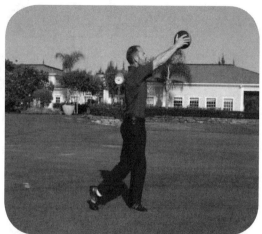

Purpose: To learn to accelerate from the ground up with the axis intact, while loading and unloading the body, and learn to create a complete and balanced finish.

Set up with a straight axis holding the ball with a loose grip and extended but not locked arms in front of the shoulders (the created triangle between the arms and shoulders stays intact). Engage the abs and rotate the shoulders and hips to the back side while sitting into your back leg. Re-engage the abs just before the turnaround and rotate to the front and upward, starting from the ground up, beginning with the legs, then hips, torso, shoulders and finally arms, while keeping a perfect axis. There should be a seamless transition at the change of direction Finish with the hips pointing toward the target, reaching up with the arms in a balanced posture with a straight but not locked knee. Feel the weight transfer from the back leg to the front leg. Avoid a reverse C by keeping the abs engaged. This exercise can also be done with the cable or rubber band.

11. RB One arm RB push

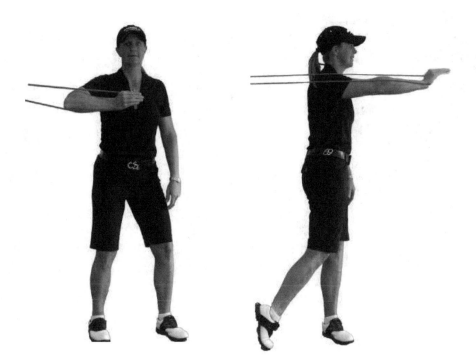

Purpose: To learn to initiate the rotation and create power with your legs and hips; learn to finish in a complete and balanced position stacked over your left leg with hips pointing toward the target.

Set up with your axis intact and hips in line with the RB. Relax arm and grip, knees slightly bent. Start by engaging the abs, initiating the rotation from the ground up, starting with the legs, then hips, torso, shoul¬ders and finally the arm. Complete the finish with the hips pointing to the target, back leg extended with gluteus engaged, upper body stacked over the straight but not locked front leg. Feel the weight as it transfers from the back leg to the front leg. Avoid falling into a "reverse C" by keeping the abs engaged.

12. Shot put

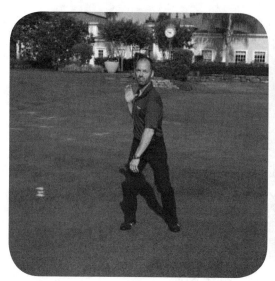 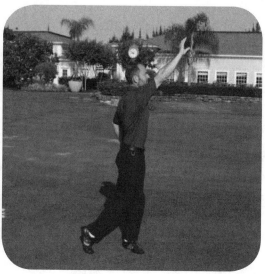

Purpose: To learn to accelerate from the ground up with the axis intact while loading and unloading the body; learn to create a complete and balanced finish.

Set up in a shot put position, sitting into the back leg to load it up while maintaining your axis. Engage the abs and initiate the acceleration and rotation from the ground up, starting with the legs, then hips, torso, shoulders and then finally the arms. Rotate to a full finish with the hips pointing toward the target, legs, upper body and arms extended, being balanced and stacked over the straight but not locked front leg (avoid a reverse C by keeping the abs engaged; do not lock the knee).

Part 5

The Workout Programs

HERE ARE THE different workout programs for the different phases. Follow these phases for the safest and most efficient way to improve your fitness and performance.

Even though some workouts are targeted around one part of the body, it is important to remember that you always want to engage the whole body in order to distribute the load through your complete system, for example, doing the Hammer Curl to Overhead, make sure you get help from your core and legs.

In the extensive list of exercises provided in this book, you will see many core exercises and some from other categories that may not show up in a particular workout. I wanted to give you enough choices and variety. Feel free to add or substitute some of them, e.g., you can add or substitute the Knee to Elbow exercise on the Arm day.

Again, these are my recommendations that have proven to be very effective with my students from beginners to pros, but sometimes it is necessary to adjust a program or some exercises to the specific needs of an individual. You can do the same if you feel that an exercise just does not agree with you. Instead, substituting a similar one may work better for you. The most important factor for your success will be that every exercise must be performed perfectly every time and that you create good consistency.

Sometimes you may not have the time or you don't feel like doing a full workout. Don't panic. Pick one of the Whole Body & Power exercises like the wood chop up and just do five to eight sets of six to eight reps apiece with good intensity. This will only take about 15 minutes and you will accomplish a lot!

The exercises that are connected with a dash are to be performed as a super-set (you just go back to back) and there is no need to have a rest in between.

1. Building and Learning

This is where you want to start — in this phase you will train your body from every angle possible and it is designed to strengthen every joint. All the stabilizing muscles and connective tissue are addressed. You also want to increase your range of motion and learn the right movement sequences. That is important in order to prepare and protect your body for the next phases as well as for competitive play. You will also learn with every exercise how to use your core to connect your body, which will give you control over your movements as well as improved strength. Some of the exercises involve smaller, single limb movements.

There are four different workout days in this phase and ideally, every week you will do two days on, followed by one day off, then two days on and two days off. That equals four workouts per week. Should it take you 10 days to get all four workouts in, that would be OK as well.

If you are new to working out with weights, start off easy for the first two rounds of the four different workouts, and gradually increase the weights as you become more comfortable with them and are sure that you are performing the exercises correctly. After the fourth week, you should reach the "heavy" resistance level with all exercises unless noted otherwise. (Some exercises can go to the maximum resistance level while oth¬ers should not exceed the medium level.)

Total time in this phase: 8 to 10 weeks

3 sets / 8 reps

[= super sets

Day 1 Arms	
1.	Twisting biceps curl – to max
2.	Triceps kickback – to max
3.	Cable concentration curl
4.	Cable triceps extension abducted
5.	Hammer curl to overhead
6.	One arm cable pull
7.	One arm cable push
8.	Crunches on PB
9.	Superman on PB

Day 2 Shoulders	
1.	DB rotation exterior up
2.	DB rotation interior up
3.	Cable rotation exterior down
4.	Cable rotation interior down
5.	DB overhead extension
6.	DB rotation neutral – to medium
7.	DB rotation abducted – to medium
8.	Straight cable rotation
9.	Obliques on PB

Day 3 Legs	
1.	Front lunge
2.	Back lunge
3.	Diagonal lunge
4.	Plié lunge
5.	DB squats
6.	Cable adductor
7.	Cable abductor
8.	Supine hip extension on PB
9.	Hamstring curl on PB

Day 4 Chest and Back	
1.	Flat bench DB chest press together – to max
2.	Bent over DB rowing
3.	Incline bench DB chest press together
4.	Standing row
5.	Pushups
6.	Pullups
7.	Wood chop down
8.	Wood chop up
9.	Plank

2. Strength

In this phase you want to gain overall strength, so more exercises will consist of full body recruitment in order to learn how to use your body as one unit. You will be using heavier weights and performing fewer reps. It is important that you have adequate rest between the single exercise sets (two to three minutes) in order to recuperate sufficiently to use enough weight for the next set.

Go to the heavy resistance level on all exercises unless noted otherwise.

Total time in this phase: 8 to 10 weeks

3 sets: 8 reps / 5 reps / 6 reps

Day 1 Arms

1.	One arm twisting biceps curl to overhead alternating (create rhythm)
2.	Cable triceps pushdown
3.	Hammer curl to overhead
4.	Rope triceps pushdown
5.	Chin ups
6.	Close grip pushup
7.	One arm cable push
8.	One arm cable pull
9.	Superman on PB

Day 2 Shoulders

1.	DB rotation exterior up alternating – to medium
2.	DB rotation interior up alternating – to medium
3.	Cable front deltoid – to medium
4.	Cable rear deltoid – to medium
5.	Lying rear deltoid – to medium
6.	Cable rotation exterior down
7.	Light power clean – to medium
8.	Hanging abs
9.	Straight cable rotation

Day 3 Chest

1.	Incline bench DB press alternating
2.	Incline BB press
3.	Pushups with weight
4.	Cable cross over
5.	Bent arm pull over – to medium
6.	Lying rope pull over
7.	Light power clean – to medium
8.	Wood chop down

Day 4 Legs

1.	Front to back lunges
2.	Plié lunges
3.	BB squats
4.	Dead lift – to medium
5.	Step up
6.	Cable abductor, adductor, front and back extension (6 reps each) - light
7.	Pushup hold rotation

KAI FUSSER

Day 5 Back

1.	Cable lat pull down
2.	Rope lat pull down alternating (create rhythm) – to medium
3.	Pullups
4.	Jockey row
5.	Kneeling two-arm lat pull down
6.	Wood chop up
7.	Prone jackknife
8.	Crunches on PB one leg

3. Power

This is a fun phase. Now you get to use your newly gained strength and add some speed to it, which will result in power. It is important that you use everything you have learned from the previous exercises: engaging the abs, body connection, power flow, movement control, etc.

Pay close attention to the release of energy, and make sure it goes to the intended target. A good warm-up is important, as speed puts extra stress on your system. Do about five to 10 minutes of light full body dynamic exercises to prepare.

It is important that you have adequate rest between the single exercise sets (two to three minutes) in order to recuperate to be able to use enough weight or produce enough power for the next set.

Total time in this phase: 5 to 6 weeks

Five sets: for all exercises, the weight ranges are described for each set for each exercise

Set 1 – 6 reps

Set 2 – 4 reps

Set 3 – 2 reps

Set 4 – 2 reps

Set 5 – 4 reps

Day 1
1. Power clean
Set 1 – medium
Set 2 – heavy
Set 3 – max
Set 4 – max
Set 5 – medium
2. Wood chop up
Set 1 – medium
Set 2 – heavy
Set 3 – max
Set 4 – max
Set 5 – medium

3. MB throw to the wall

All sets 6 to 10 lbs.

Emphasize on building power from the ground up as well as a strong release.

4. Jumping front to back lunges

All sets light to medium. Emphasis on good, trampoline-like rebounds while maintaining good rhythm.

5. One arm cable pull

Light to medium weight only. Fast rhythm

Day 2
1. Squat
Set 1 – medium
Set 2 – heavy
Set 3 – max
Set 4 – max
Set 5 – medium
2. Pushups
Set 1 – medium
Set 2 – heavy
Set 3 – max
Set 4 – max
Set 5 – medium

3. Bench jump

All sets light to medium. Concentrate on explosiveness while using the whole body.

4. MB slam to the ground

All sets six to 10 lbs. Concentrate on drawing the arms and legs together by engaging the abs just before the downward motion for the slam.

5. One arm cable push

Light to medium weight only. Fast rhythm.

Day 3
1. Dead lift
Set 1 – medium
Set 2 – heavy
Set 3 – max
Set 4 – max
Set 5 – medium
2. Wood chop down
Set 1 – medium
Set 2 – heavy
Set 3 – max
Set 4 – max
Set 5 – medium
3. Pull ups
Set 1 – medium
Set 2 – heavy
Set 3 – max
Set 4 – max
Set 5 – medium

4. Shot put

Light to medium weight only. Fast rhythm.

5. Straight cable rotation

Light to medium weight only. Fast rhythm.

4. In Season

All the gains you have made while progressing through the different phases need to be retained for as long as possible so you can utilize them during your playing season. There are different challenges during the season: time, fatigue, travelling, lack of gyms or equipment, to name just a few.

It is easy to get all caught up in just playing and practicing during that time and start neglecting your body, but that will lead to losing the physical advantage you've worked so hard to gain. The solution to this is learning how to appropriately schedule your activities during your tournament week and realizing that the workouts, rather than being in the way and adding to your commitments, will help you to perform well.

Don't be afraid that the workouts will make you too tired to play. Now that you have progressed through all your phases, your body is used to the workout stress, and it will not hamper you.

Annika would always make sure she would get three to four full workouts in during a tournament week. Many times we would do a full workout mere hours before her tee time. It set her body up to perform and, also, being a little fatigued before the round may have helped with her rhythm, taking the edge off a little. It was also a good escape for her, time away from the course and all the action.

It is important during that time that you keep the workouts short and concentrated with the appropriate intensity. The best way to find out how your body (or mind) will react after a workout is to try it with your practice rounds. Work out at different times beforehand and then go out and play and see how you feel and how you perform. This will also give you the confidence that a workout will not hinder your play but, in fact, help it.

Three workouts a week is an ideal goal but, if you miss one in a week, don't stress over it.

These workouts include full body exercises, which require high coordination. Here, too, you can substitute an exercise if you feel the need. There are fewer exercises and fewer reps, therefore, you want to keep the intensity up. The complete workout should not take more than 30 to 45 minutes. The exercises are also mixed body parts so you should not get overly fatigued or sore in one particular area. Should you have a week where the playing schedule is just too crazy, you can always shorten the workouts to two or three exercises. Even if you don't work out for one week, it should not be a problem. Just don't let it become a habit.

Unless noted, go to "heavy" weight with all the exercises. You can pick one exercise in each workout to go to maximum weight and intensity. The rotational exercises will be done at medium level.

3 sets: 8 reps / 5 reps / 5 reps

Day 1
1. Incline bench DB chest press alternating
2. Pushups
3. Power clean
4. Obliques on PB with MB
5. One arm cable pull: 1st set medium – 2nd set heavy – 3rd set light with speed (8 to 10 reps)
6. Wood chop down: 1st set medium – 2nd set heavy – 3rd set light with speed (8 to 10 reps)

Day 2
1. Cable lat pull down
2. Pull ups
3. Deadlift
4. Pushup hold rotation: 1st set medium – 2nd set heavy – 3rd set light with speed (8 to 10 reps)
5. Wood chop up: 1st set medium – 2nd set heavy – 3rd set light with speed (8 to 10 reps)

Day 3
1. Front to back lunges
2. Bench jump
3. BB squats
4. Knee to elbow
5. Shot put: 1st set medium – 2nd set heavy – 3rd set light with speed (8 to 10 reps)
6. Straight cable rotation: 1st set medium – 2nd set heavy – 3rd set light with speed (8 to 10 reps)

5. Travel and no Gym

These are workouts you can throw in anytime or anywhere, they are great for when you are out on the road or even at home when you don't have time to go to the gym. They are designed to be done with a minimal amount of equipment, keep them short and intense to get the most out of them. When travelling it is easy to just take along some small equipment like some runner band and a jump rope.

These are just some samples. You can take many of the exercises in this book and put them into one of these workouts. Be inventive with the exercises, for example, a squat can be done slow, fast, or with a wide, narrow, or close stance, and with or without a rubber band. As efficient as these workouts are, you will never again have any excuse not to work out. Three of these workouts a week are ideal but even doing just two a week will put you ahead of the game.

Use rubber bands to increase resistance and adjust the intensity by adding speed or taking away stability.

3 sets / 8-10 reps

Day 1
1. Front to back lunge
2. Plié lunges
3. Squats
4. Ab scissors
5. Side plank
6. Pushup rotation with reach through
7. Sprints in place (4 minutes HIIT)

Day 2
1. Pushup wide grip
2. RB chest press
3. Pushup close grip
4. RB push
5. Knee to elbow
6. Plank
7. Get ups (three sets of 8, each side)

Day 3
1. RB twisting curl to overhead
2. RB triceps kickback
3. RB pull
4. RB straight rotation
5. RB shot put
6. Jumping front to back lunges
7. Pushup to jump (three sets of 8)

Recommended Reading and Websites

1. Annika Sorenstam, *Golf Annika's Way*

2. Dr. Michael Colgan, *The New Power Program and many other of his publications*

3. Paul Check, *Golf Biomechanic's Manual and many of his publications*

4. Mark Verstegen, *many of his publications*

5. Juan Carlos Santana, *Functional Training Companion Guide and many other of his publications*

6. Robert E. McAtee and Jeff Charland, *Facilitated Stretching*

7. Mike Boyle, *Foam Roll Techniques DVD*

8. Gray Cook, *Movement*

9. Chuck Wolf, *Flexibility Highways in Motion DVD*

10. Gregg Cochlan, *Love Leadership*

11. Gregg Cochlan and Ron Medved, *World Peace "Really"*

12. Michael Pollan, *In Defense of Food*

13. William Wolcott and Trish Fahey, *The Metabolic Typing Diet*

14. David Bodanis, *E=mc(2)*

15. www.kaifusser.com

16. www.fusserfitnessandnutrition.com

17. www.TheAnnikaAacademy.com

18. www.ThePacificInstitute.com

KAI FUSSER

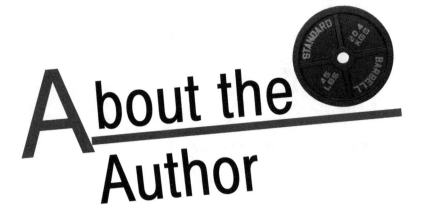

About the Author

Kai Fusser, M.S. (Dipl. Ing.)

KAI FUSSER WAS born in 1963 in Germany and holds a master's degree in nautical engineering from the University of Oldenburg in Germany.

Fusser's knowledge and experience gained through training superb athletes, such as Annika Sorenstam, Grant Hill, Darin Shapiro and others, is incalculable. He has been involved in professional sports since 1985, first as a competitive waterskier, and then as a coach and trainer in waterskiing and wake boarding. In 2001, Fusser implemented his workout philosophy to train Annika Sorenstam. During that time, Annika gained in excess of 25 yards of additional driving distance while simultaneously improving accuracy. Annika was then voted Female Athlete of the Year twice in a row.

Fusser currently trains more than 15 LPGA and PGA players as well as many junior and collegiate players. Cumulatively, his players have won 13 major championships and over 110 tournaments on the LPGA, Ladies and Mens European Tour, Japanese LPGA and PGA. His waterskiers and wake boarders have won over 100 titles among them, including multiple X-Games and Gravity-Games.

Fusser is a certified facilitator for The Pacific Institute's *Investment in Excellence* course, geared to develop the right attitude for success through cognitive psychology. Fusser has been invited to share and teach his program at numerous universities and expert summits and is a frequent lecturer at the TPI World Fitness Summit. Fusser has been featured in many media outlets like *GOLF*

Magazine, *GolfWorld*, Japan's *Golf Digest*, Germany's *Golf Journal*, *Golf Fitness Magazine*, *Waterski* Magazine, ESPN, *USA Today*, 60 Minutes, the Golf Channel and more.

Fusser's workouts revolve around the philosophy, "Efficiency through perfect movement." All training is performed with functional exercises, ideally utilizing the whole body without isolating any body part. Therefore, no machines are used; instead, the exercises are performed via dumbbells, barbells, cable crossover, medicine balls, gym balls and calisthenics. The workouts are designed to improve and maximize strength, power, balance, flexibility and endurance, building and utilizing core strength, and developing a good base from which to work in order to rotate around the body's axis. Fusser notes that, as everybody's build is different, he teaches the most efficient way for that particular individual to move to maximize one's performance at any level, whether they are a weekend warrior or a top professional athlete. He also teaches "power flow," his unique method to encourage forces to flow through the body to be evenly distributed, thereby reducing stress on individual body parts and joints, the foundation for injury prevention, while maximizing efficiency of movement.

Kai is currently the Director of Fitness at the prestigious Annika Academy in Orlando, Florida.

KAI FUSSER

Index

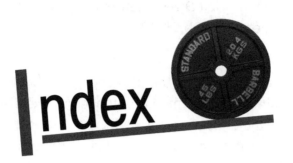

KAI FUSSER

EXERCISES

WEIGHT TRAINING FOR GOLF

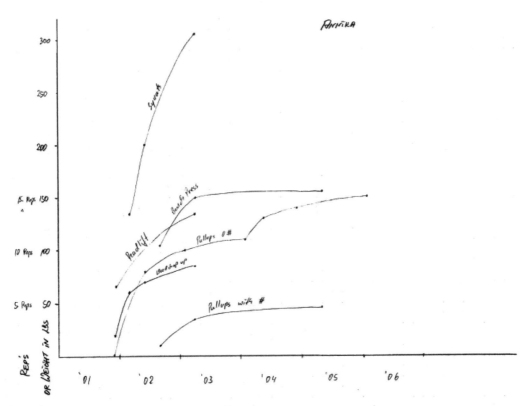

I made up this chart in 2005, it shows Annika's progress in the gym over 3,5 years. Note the pullups with and without weight, the squats from 135 to 305 pounds.

KAI FUSSER

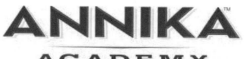

Kai Fusser, M.S.
"Efficiency through perfect movement"

Name_____ Day_____
Sets_____   Reps_____

WEIGHT TRAINING FOR GOLF

EXERCISES	Date								
	wgt.								
	reps								
	wgt.								
	reps								
	wgt								
	reps								
	wgt								
	reps								
	wgt								
	reps								
	wgt								
	reps								
	wgt								
	reps								
	wgt								
	reps								
	wgt								
	reps								
	wgt								
	reps								

Track your results with this sample training log.

Kai Fusser, M.S.
Orlando, FL
407-758-5961
The Power Program To Optimum Strength and Health

Arnika

Day ___I___

Sets ___5___ Reps 8/6/4/4

TRAINING LOG

EXERCISES		Home 6-17-04	Home 6-23	Boston 6-28	Tahoe 7-12	Evian 7-20	England 7-26	Orlando 8-19	Orlando 8-23		
1. Standing Barbell Lyes	wgt.	45/8/10/10/10	45/10/10/10	45/15/15	45/45/15/15	DG 49 12/12/2	45/45/15/15	45/45/6/15	45/15/15		
	reps.	8/8/6/6	8/8/6/6	8/8/6/8	8/8/6/8	8/8/3	8/8/3/8	6/8/8	8/8/6/6		
2. Power clean / Squat to overhead	wgt.	45/55/55/55	45/55/55	45/55/5/55	45/55/55/55	45/45/45	45/45/45	45/45/45	45/45/45		
	reps.	8/6/6/6	8/6/6	8/6/6	8/6/6	8/8/8	8/8/8	8/8/8	8/8/8		
3. Pushups w. Hands on Ball / Feet on bench	wgt.	0/0/0/0	0/0/0/0	0/0/0/0	0/0/0/0	0/0/0	0/0/0	0/0/0	0/0/10		
	reps.	8/8/4/4	8/4/4	8/4/4/4	8/4/4/4	4/4/4 4/4/4	8/4/4	4/4/4 4/4/4	5/5/4 5/5/4		
4. Two Arm Front PB Rotation	wgt.	46/7				1/2/2 49	2/3/3 49	5/6/7	5/7/10		
	reps.	8/8/8				8/8/8	8/8/8	8/8/8	8/8/8		
5. Front Hipsquat	wgt.	25/8/30	25/30/35	25/35/35	25/35/35	25/25/25	25/30/35	30/35/35	30/35/37		
	reps.	8/8/6	8/8/8	8/8/8	8/8/8	8/8/8	8/8/8	8/8/8	8/8/8		
6. Rotational Crunches with Med. Ball on ball	wgt.	0/0/0			4/6/6			6/6/6	6/6/6		
	reps.	8/8/8 8/8/2			8/10/10 8/10/10		8/8	8/6/6	8/8/8		
7. Prone Leg Scissors o. Ball (Roll on arms then to under chest)	wgt.	0/0/0	0/0/0	0/0/0	0/0/0	0/0/0	0/0	0/0/0	0/0/0		
	reps.	8/8/4/4	8/8/4/4	8/4/4/4	8/4/4/4	8/8/8	8/4	8/4/4/4	4/4/4		
	wgt.										
	reps.										
	wgt.										
	reps.										
	wgt.										
	reps.										

KAI FUSSER

** No copies of this written program without permission

We were very stringent on record keeping, I still have most every workout sheet from the start in 2001. Here you see a training log for day 1 of an in season program. Note the locations on the top, Home (Orlando), Boston, Tahoe, Evian (Evian Masters), England (British Open), Orlando.

WEIGHT TRAINING FOR GOLF

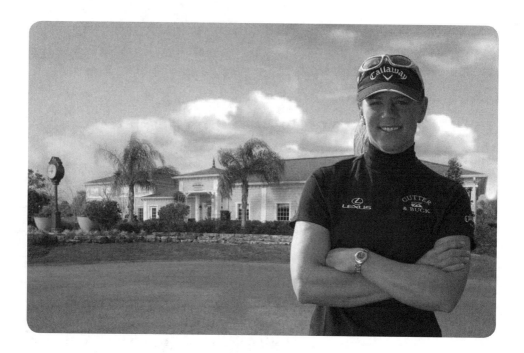

ANNIKA™
ACADEMY

ANNIKA Academy is a state-of-the-art, "boutique" teaching facility housed at Reunion Resort, outside of Orlando, Florida. The Academy opened in August 2006 as a way to share Annika's passion for golf and fitness, along with her personal swing coach Henri Reis, personal trainer Kai Fusser and sister Charlotta. Their simple techniques allow players of all skill levels to reach their potential by transferring more energy and power to the golf course. The ANNIKA Academy is a Certified Callaway Performance Center with two spacious hitting booths that offer custom club fitting and video swing analysis. The Academy provides individual instruction, personalized fitness and nutrition programs and custom corporate packages. Guests can play with Annika or learn the proven methods from the coaches who guided her legendary career.

"Share My Passion"

www.theannikaacademy.com